Competency-Based Nursing Education

Guide to Achieving Outstanding Learner Outcomes

Marion G. Anema, PhD, RN, has held faculty appointments at a variety of educational institutions, including most recently: Associate Director, Nursing Programs, College of Health Professions, Western Governors University; Mentor and Faculty Chair, Walden University; Dean, School of Nursing, Tennessee State University; and Assistant Dean, Texas Woman's University, Dallas. Dr. Anema is currently a consultant developing online nursing programs at MidAmerica Learning in Abilene, Texas. She holds certificates as an online instructor in case management, online quality management, and intensive bioethics (Georgetown University). Her scholarly articles have been published in *Dimensions of Critical Care Nursing,* the *Journal of Nursing Administration, Nursing,* the *Journal of Nursing Education, Nurse Educator, International Nursing Review, Computers in Nursing,* and the *Journal of Continuing Education in Nursing,* among others.

Jan McCoy, PhD, RN, has been a school nurse, flight nurse, and cardiac catheterization lab nurse. For the major part of her nursing career she held appointments at Central Wyoming College. At Central Wyoming College, she was a member of the nursing faculty; Nursing Program Director; Division Chair, Professional/Technical Division, and Allied Health Division; and Director of Distance Education/Lifelong Learning. More recently, Dr. McCoy has served as a nursing faculty member at Walden University; Individual Service Coordinator, Wyoming Department of Health; and Independent Contractor and Consultant for Sylvan Learning Systems; as well as interim Director of Nursing Programs and Mentor at Western Governors University, Salt Lake City, Utah. Dr. McCoy continues to offer consulting services for nursing programs involved in curriculum development/revision and/or program accreditation processes. She holds an online instructor certificate from Walden University and was awarded a Kellogg Fellowship through the University of Portland.

Competency-Based Nursing Education

Guide to Achieving Outstanding Learner Outcomes

Marion G. Anema, PhD, RN
Jan McCoy, PhD, RN

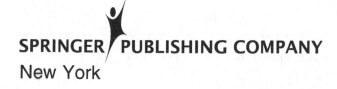

SPRINGER PUBLISHING COMPANY

New York

Springer Publishing Company, LLC
11 West 42nd Street
New York, NY 10036
www.springerpub.com

Acquisitions Editor: Margaret Zuccarini
Project Manager: Pamela Lankas
Cover design: Bill Smith Studios
Composition: International Graphic Services

E-book ISBN: 978-0826-1-0510-3

10 11 12 13/ 5 4 3 2 1

The authors and the publisher of this Work have made every effort to use sources believed to be reliable to provide information that is accurate and compatible with the standards generally accepted at the time of publication. Because medical science is continually advancing, our knowledge base continues to expand. Therefore, as new information becomes available, changes in procedures become necessary. We recommend that the reader always consult current research and specific institutional policies before performing any clinical procedure. The authors and publisher shall not be liable for any special, consequential, or exemplary damages resulting, in whole or in part, from the readers' use of, or reliance on, the information contained in this book. The publisher has no responsibility for the persistence or accuracy of URLs for external or third-party Internet Web sites referred to in this publication and does not guarantee that any content on such Web sites is, or will remain, accurate or appropriate.

Library of Congress Cataloging-in-Publication Data

Anema, Marion G.
    Competency-based nursing education : guide to achieving outstanding learner outcomes / Marion G. Anema, Jan McCoy, authors.
        p. ; cm.
    Includes bibliographical references and index.
    ISBN 978-0-8261-0509-7 (alk. paper)
    1. Nursing—Study and teaching. 2. Competency-based education. I. McCoy, Jan. II. Title. [DNLM: 1. Education, Nursing—methods. 2. Competency-Based Education. WY 18 A579c 2009]
    RT71.A555 2009
    610.73076—dc22
                                        2009035610

Printed in the United States of America by the Hamilton Printing Company

To Carrie B. Lenburg, EdD, RN, FAAN, who, in the 1990s, challenged the nursing and health professions to adopt competency-based education, and to educators everywhere who are dedicated to the use of competency-based education to achieve outstanding learner outcomes.

Contents

Preface

The inspiration for this book came from our experiences as nurses providing direct care to patients, serving as advanced practice nurses, supervising nursing students, listening to the needs of our clinical colleagues, and from opportunities we have had to revise and develop new programs.

The need for competency-based education (CBE) has been recognized for years. The preparation of graduates for a wide range of professions and trades has been a concern of employers. Education and work were disconnected and new graduates did not have the basic skills to function in the workplace. Students were weak in universal skills such as reading, writing, oral communication, mathematical computations, creative thinking, problem solving, managing self, working with groups, and working effectively within an organization. Additionally, graduates needed specific, entry-level skills to function in their specific disciplines.

The health-related professions require demonstrated competency in their practitioners. New graduates need to function at a specific beginning level to provide safe care. Continuing competency is also required to ensure that expert, quality care is being provided. Leaders in medical education programs have been at the forefront of implementing CBE approaches. Carrie Lenburg is the nursing leader who developed a model and framework for CBE. The public, regulatory agencies, and professional organizations require accountability from educational institutions and programs. CBE provides a way to help ensure that learners are competent at the end of educational endeavors.

This book is designed as a resource for nurses and health professionals in all disciplines who are responsible for diverse education programs. The book is unique because it brings together all the elements of CBE and provides a road map for developing, implementing, and evaluating competency-based approaches to education.

Chapter 1 includes an overview of CBE with foundational information about the driving forces that support it. Chapter 2 focuses on the essential elements of CBE and addresses the question, "Why should we have CBE programs?" Different models are presented and the Lenburg model is used to communicate how to develop a CBE course or program. Chapter 3 provides an overview of the processes essential to implementing a CBE program. The principles of adult education, active and interactive learning, and demonstration of competency at the end of an instructional course or program are addressed.

Chapter 4 focuses on the development of competency statements that address the needs of different learners: patients and consumers, professional staff, and students in formal academic programs. Current standards of practice, regulatory requirements, and employer and consumer expectations and their use for CBE are explained. The processes for creating learning statements/activities for objective and performance assessment are included.

Chapter 5 includes the specific steps for developing both objective and performance assessments required to measure outcome competencies. This chapter reviews reliability and validity processes to help ensure high-quality assessment tools. Chapter 6 concentrates on gathering individual assessment information, aggregating it, and organizing it for program or course outcome assessments. Combining or aggregating individual outcome data provides the big picture of what is happening in a course or program.

The final chapter addresses why CBE is so important if educational outcomes are going to meet the needs of learners, graduates, employers, and organizations. The challenges of implementing CBE are addressed. Strategies and suggestions, based on theories selected to support success, are presented. There is an activity at the end of each chapter that guides readers through the steps in using CBE. Additional resources provide further information about CBE.

The book challenges readers to reconsider what they are currently doing in their educational programs and to revise or construct new approaches to ensuring that learners are competent. The processes for implementing CBE can start with one learning module, one course, or the revision of an entire program, as needed.

1 Vision of Competency-Based Education

MARION G. ANEMA

OVERVIEW

This chapter provides an overview, definition, and exploration of competency-based education (CBE). The terms *competence*, *competency*, and *performance*, although similar, have differences in meaning that cause confusion. A variety of approaches are used to develop CBE programs, curricula, or courses. External regulatory agencies and accrediting organizations, such as the regional and specialized accrediting bodies for all levels of formal education, as well as the professional and discipline-specialty organizations, all have their own standards. The Joint Commission on Accreditation of Healthcare Organizations (JCAHO) coupled with the ability of patient care organizations to achieve Magnet status are drivers for using a competency-based approach to demonstrate outcomes. Connecting the different stakeholders is necessary to ensure that graduates entering their professions are competent to function in complex, changing work environments. A focus on the health of the general public emphasizes the importance of measuring outcomes of programs designed to prevent disease and maintain health.

This chapter provides references and links to be used as additional resources that support and expand the information presented. The activities (found at the end of the chapter) provide a structure for determining why a change is needed in an organization. The following chapters build on the information in this chapter concerning CBE.

INTRODUCTION

There is a quiet revolution at work in education that started over 25 years ago. New directions for learning are being advocated in all levels and types of education. Institutions face increasing amounts of information, new technologies are introduced, funding is decreasing, and there are external demands for accountability (Evers, Rush, & Berdrow, 1998). A major focus is a competency-based approach to all levels and types of education: K–12, undergraduate, graduate, continuing education and training in the workplace, and patient and consumer programs.

Diploma- and degree-granting institutions, employer training programs, individual professionals, and diverse educational programs are all facing the same issues. The cost of providing educational offerings continues to increase. Students complete educational programs that do not prepare them to function in the workplace or prepare them for the next level of education. For example, postsecondary institutions keep adding courses, tutorials, and other remedial or developmental offerings to help students be successful in their new learning environments. New employees cannot meet job requirements. Professionals must meet relicensure requirements. Organizations and institutions must also meet external approval and accreditation guidelines. The major problem is the lack of data and evidence on the educational outcomes. A great deal of time, effort, and resources are spent to provide all these different educational programs without achieving positive results. CBE can contribute to making a difference in preparing new graduates and current workers to function effectively in their jobs.

All over the world, education is being conceptualized and delivered in new ways. Technology, in many different forms, has transformed education by providing broader access and the ability to collect and manage data to assess outcomes. Beyond colleges and universities, organizations have adopted performance-based learning developed from specific competencies. Adult learners have different needs and expectations for their educational experiences. Distance-education options have increased access for adult learners. Students enter educational programs with specific competencies. The competency-based approach to education addresses accountability for educational outcomes and aligns workforce needs, employers, job expectations, and the assessment of competence in educational programs.

Colleges and universities have been slow to adopt new approaches such as CBE. Today, educational outcomes in higher education institutions generally focus on what is produced. The measures used help institutions demonstrate accountability to internal and external stakeholders, based on retention, graduation, and placement rates (Voorhees, 2001). These measures do not directly determine what students know and are able to do in work settings. A simple definition of a CBE approach is that assessments ensure that graduates in all disciplines have the essential knowledge, skills, and attitudes to enter the workforce and begin functioning in entry-level positions.

There are several reasons for the current interest in CBE:

1. Educational institutions and providers need evidence that anyone who completes a degree or course has achieved a required level of competency.
2. Accrediting, regulatory, and professional groups want assurance that completion of an educational endeavor indicates competency.
3. There is greater accountability for the costs and time it takes to complete educational endeavors and determine if they achieve the expected outcomes.
4. Employers hire new workers who do not have basic competencies required for entry-level positions.
5. Employers invest in extensive training programs to address the initial needs of new employees and the continuing training needs of all employees, especially those in complex, changing work environments.
6. Regulatory, legal, external standards, and quality measures require demonstration of competence.
7. Workers need to continue their own personal and professional development to advance their careers and make positive contributions to organizations.

The following are examples of initiatives that drew attention to CBE and provided a foundation for implementation:

1. The creation of the National Skills Standard Board in the United States to develop a national system of skills standards (Voorhees, 2001).
2. The Dearing Report (1997) addressed the issues of lifelong learning and portability of skills in the United Kingdom.
3. In Australia, competencies and skills standards are part of subuniversity programs (Faris, 1995).
4. The United States has adopted competency-based approaches in K–12 education.
5. Kerka (1998) observed that competency standards are related to meeting global competition and accountability. Such initiatives are seen in Britain, Australia, New Zealand, and the United States.
6. Employers support and require certifications related to specific jobs.

A challenge in beginning CBE efforts was to conceptualize and define what competency means and then translate it into useful and meaningful language.

CONCEPTUALIZING COMPETENCE

It is valuable to realize that there are different approaches to conceptualizing competence. This is important as institutions start to implement CBE curricula because the mission, philosophy, and goals of the entities need to be met. Gonczi (1994) described three ways of conceptualizing competence:

1. A behaviorist or task-specific approach that is assessed by observation or performance for evidence.
2. An attribute or generic-skills approach and general attributes that are crucial to effective performance, based on general competences already learned.
3. An integrated or task–attribute approach.

Juceviciene and Lepaite (2005) proposed a multidisciplinary approach to the conceptualization of competence. They viewed performance as having different hierarchical levels that require different levels of competence:

1. Level 1: Behavior competencies relate to operational work performance and have to meet the demands of the workplace. They have clearly stated constituent parts, consisting of competencies.
2. Level 2: Added competencies based on behavior and additional knowledge needed to improve work.
3. Level 3: Integrated competencies that support change of internal and external working conditions. Knowledge, skills, and understanding are integrated into internal and external work conditions.
4. Level 4: Holistic competencies necessary to develop new work and transfer knowledge and skills to new situations.

Each organization or group will have to consider various concepts of competency to determine a fit with its mission, goals, and philosophy. A further area of ambiguity concerns the difference among competence, competency, and performance.

Competency, Competence, and Performance

Competency focuses on an individual's ability to perform activities related to work, life skills, or learning. *Competence* describes actions or skills the person should be able to demonstrate. While (1994) makes an important distinction between the concepts of "competence" and "performance." She recognized that competence is concerned with perceived skills and cannot be directly measured. *Performance* relates to specific behaviors that are measurable and can reflect what workers actually do.

Eraut (1998) reviewed literature and found distinctions between competency (specific sets of skills) and competence (an individual's general capability to carry out his/her job). Xu, Xu, and Zhang (2001) studied this issue and completed a study to determine whether there are differences between the two concepts. The results suggested that competence is job-related and refers to a person's ability to meet those requirements. Competency is person-related and refers to a person's knowledge, skills, and abilities that make it possible to effectively function in a job. It is clear that definitions of competence and performance are very similar and cause confusion between (Watson, Stimpson, Topping, & Porock, 2002). For instance, Worth-Butler, Murphy, and Fraser (1994), and Norman, Watson, Murrells, Calman, and Redfern (2000) have suggested that concepts of performance and competence are inseparable.

Eraut (1994) and Gonczi (1994) have different perspectives and are convinced that competence integrates attributes with performance. Girot (1993), supported by Bradshaw (1997, 1998), who highlighted the uncertainty in the definition of competence, went on to discuss the problems caused by such a situation and made a number of recommendations regarding the assessment of the competence of nurses and others. Differences in explanations about competency lead to a discussion of the definition of the term.

Definitions of Competency

The word *competency* is widely used in education, but there is no common understanding of what it means in actual educational settings. Researchers and scholars attach different meanings and provide diverse examples of how to implement and assess CBE systems. Watson, Stimpson, Topping, and Porock (2002) reviewed 61 articles related to competency in nursing education and found that in 22 of the articles, the term *competency* was not defined.

According to Tilley (2008), a clear and accepted definition of competency does not exist across nursing education and practice. Although competency is defined in different ways, there is a common goal; to ensure nurses have the knowledge, skills, and abilities expected and required for their practice settings.

The word *competent* is derived from Latin and means having essential qualities and abilities to function in specific ways. The National Council of State Boards of Nursing (2005) describes competency as the ability to apply knowledge and interpersonal, decision-making, and psychomotor skills to nursing practice roles

A problem with the lack of clarity and common understanding is that CBE is implemented with only selected elements or is competency-based in name only. Even with a range of definitions, there is some general agreement about the characteristics of CBE. They include:

1. Acquisition of essential cognitive, psychomotor, and affective skills;
2. Continued development of skills;
3. Broadly based competency development derived from the best professional evidence, current standards, and regulations;
4. Authentic assessments which are valid and reliable;
5. The use of adult learning principles;
6. Individual learning styles and abilities are recognized and appreciated.

In spite of the differences in and ambiguity about the terms, there is concern about the preparation of all graduates and, in particular, concern about graduates of nursing and other health-related programs. Employers who are hiring new graduates raise the following concerns related to postsecondary education and employability:

1. Degrees signify competence only in a major,
2. Competency focuses on the cognitive and knowledge levels,
3. The application level may be weak,
4. Specific competencies are not identified and included in curricula,
5. College transcripts list course titles rather than specific competencies,
6. Graduates do not highlight general and specific competencies in their resumes and interviews,
7. Graduates do not share specific examples of how the competencies were developed (Voorhees, 2001).

Many panels and commissions have identified and shared lists of foundational and advanced competencies. They generally include:

1. Basic skills (reading, writing, mathematics, speaking, and listening);
2. Thinking skills (thinking creatively, decision making, problem solving);
3. Personal qualities (individual responsibility, self-esteem, social skills, managing self, and integrity) (Voorhees, 2001);
4. Four base competencies, determined by Evers, Rush, and Berdrow (1998) (managing self, communicating, organizing innovation, and managing change).

Table 1.1

SUMMARY OF 21st-CENTURY WORKPLACE SKILLS			
ATTITUDES AND PERSONAL CHARACTERISTICS	ESSENTIAL SKILLS	INTEGRATIVE-APPLIED SKILLS	PREMIUM SKILLS
Adaptability, flexibility, resiliency, accept ambiguity	Competency skills for simple tasks	Application of technology to tasks	Ability to understand organizational and contextual issues
Creativity	Interpersonal skills, team skills	Critical thinking	Ethics
Empathy	Numeracy and computation skills at the ninth-grade level	Customer contact skills	Foreign-language fluency
Positive attitude, good work ethic, ability to self-manage	Reading at the ninth-grade level	Information user skills	Globalism, internationalization skills
Reliability, dependability	Speaking and listening	Presentation skills	Multicultural competence skills
Responsibility, honesty, integrity	Writing	Problem recognition, definition, solution formation	Negotiation skills
		Reasoning	Project management and supervision
			Systems thinking

Sets of general or foundational skills (competencies) have been identified and the need for discipline-specific competencies has been addressed. Voorhees (2001) proposed a list of 21st-century workplace skills. They fall into four major categories related to the general education and liberal arts portions of degree requirements and programs. They are summarized in Table 1.1.

Most postsecondary school graduates need the skills proposed in Table 1.1 to survive and thrive in 21st-century workplaces. The business and industry communities do not want to dictate curricula and programs but do want a voice in finding ways to better prepare graduates. Promoting collaboration between educators and workplaces is one way to make improvements.

Nagelsmith (1995) describes the basis of professional competence as a set of essential and relevant knowledge, skills, and attitudes. There are different elements needed to achieve competency:

1. Determination of knowledge, skills, and abilities required for graduates of nursing education programs, based on standards and legal requirements.
2. Relevance to current practice.
3. Registration and licensing examinations by boards of nursing.
4. Board of nursing continuing education requirements for licensing.
5. Employer monitoring of required staff development modules, completion of courses, demonstrations, and examinations.
6. Certification requirements by professional nursing organizations.
7. Standards and accreditation for nursing practice guidelines.

There is consensus among many groups that nursing and other health care graduates are not prepared to function in complex work environments. CBE is especially important in health-related programs. It is essential that providers of all types of health care and services are competent to carry out their roles. Health professions promise competency and have diverse methods to measure it. Since the late 1990s, external groups, such as the Citizen Advocacy Center (2006) and the Pew Health Professions Commission Taskforce on Health Care Workforce Regulation (1998), began to question if the existing processes truly assured competency. Consumers and groups interested in health policy were concerned about patient safety and effectiveness of the health care workforce.

Concerns related to the competency of new health professionals, including nurses, are:

1. A significant number of new nursing graduates do not become registered. The NCLEX-RN examination results for 2008 show that 87.3% of first-time U.S.-educated nurses passed the first time. When graduates repeated the examination, only 53.4%

passed. For internationally educated nurses, the first-time pass rate was 45.6%, and for repeated attempts was 24.5%. The overall pass rate was 72.4% (National Council of State Boards of Nursing, 2008).

2. In the United States, there are no uniform processes among the states to assess the continued competence of registered nurses. Wendt and Marks (2007) completed the first comprehensive study on a national level to determine if there is a core set of competencies that can be used to assess nurses in all practice settings and with a wide range of experience.

3. The Performance-Based Development System (PBDS) has been used in more than 350 health care agencies in 46 states to assess nurses' critical thinking and interpersonal skills abilities. Findings indicate that 65% to 76% of inexperienced RNs do not meet expectations for entry-level clinical judgment ability (del Bruno, 2005).

4. The National Academies stated that there are no links among accreditation, certification, and license requirements and identified five core competencies that all health professionals should have for the 21st century (Griener & Knebel, 2003).

5. The Pew Commission (1998) proposed 25 competencies for health care professionals.

Although there is common ground about what is needed to better prepare graduates for work, as well as assure their continuing competence, there are differing views about the approaches, benefits, and value of CBE systems. Table 1.2 summarizes several issues and concerns related to competency of new graduates from health-related programs.

Approaches to Competency-Based Education

Although there are different perspectives on the definition of CBE, diverse groups see the need to incorporate common elements:

1. Consumers, regulatory, educational, and practice groups establish partnerships.

2. Collaboration and innovation in education and practice settings support the development and maintenance of competent workforce (Coonan, 2008).

Table 1.2

ISSUES/CONCERNS RELATED TO NEW GRADUATES OF HEALTH PROGRAMS

CONCERNS	ASSESSMENTS	GOALS
Freshman college students fail required composition paper that is at a 12th-grade level.	Results of student papers indicate that 90% of the students make major errors in grammar, logical progression of ideas, and citing sources.	90% of the students have minimal errors in the three areas.
New registered nurses are unable to recognize signs and symptoms that indicate problems in hospitalized patients diagnosed with myocardial infarction.	Patient records indicate nurses do chart signs and symptoms, but 50% did not carry out appropriate nursing actions, based on best evidence and standards of practice.	90% of new registered nurses will carry out appropriate nursing actions.
Senior nursing students fail a critical unit exam in their advanced medical/surgical nursing course. They pass the course because of higher grades on the other unit exams.	70% of senior nursing students fail the neurology unit exam and have not demonstrated a minimum level of knowledge in this area.	100% of the students will pass the neurology unit exam with a minimum grade of 80%.
Persons diagnosed with diabetes are required to complete educational program and modules related to all aspects of managing their condition.	80% of the persons attending the program complete the medication and diet modules and 50% complete the exercise and managing life with diabetes modules.	100% of the persons attending the course will complete all the modules.
The staff and parents of elementary school age children are concerned about potential obesity, the food served at school, and lack of exercise. Students do have health classes where these topics are covered.	Data were collected related to these areas. It was determined that 60% of the children are overweight, school menus do not meet American Dietetics Association nutritional guidelines, and children only participate in physical education twice a week for 30 minutes.	Data will be collected in three areas to determine changes in the students' health related to weight, eating habits, and activities. The desired outcomes and all results are within normal limits or guidelines.

3. Educational systems respond to changes in complex work environments (Coonan, 2008).
4. Learners have an active role in determining their educational needs.
5. The primary focus is on identifying and measuring specific learning outcomes for initial and continued competence.
6. Required competencies include all the domains required for practice in a discipline.
7. Assessments are given at each level with the learners demonstrating competence at each level.
8. Assessments are done at different points in time, using a variety of approaches.

Fitness for practice or competency in an area is congruent with the completion of an educational program. Although there is agreement among supporters of CBE, who see the value and benefits, there are also opposing views.

Differing Views of CBE

According to Voorhees (2001), institutions of higher education are recognizing that institutional accountability, articulation and student transfer concerns, and employability issues are reasons for considering movement to CBE. The value and benefits of a competency-based approach include:

1. Applicability at the course, program, institutional, and system levels.
2. Participation of internal and external stakeholders in determining the desired knowledge, skills, attitudes, and dispositions important in diverse work settings.
3. Developing assessments derived from specific competencies.
4. Support for the development of learning experiences and assignments that help students become proficient in the competencies essential to different disciplines and settings (U.S. Department of Education, 2006).

Opponents of CBE primarily in higher education, raise the following issues for not implementing change:

1. General resistance to change in colleges and universities.
2. Higher education should not be totally aligned with employer and other external stakeholders demands.
3. CBE is currently viewed as being useful primarily in vocational or technical education settings.
4. Applying CBE to general and liberal education is reductionist and prescriptive.
5. The faculty currently determines assessments based on professional judgment, and CBE shifts this process to include others (Voorhees, 2001).
6. Lack of emphasis on CBE in programs that prepare educators.
7. The need to train educators to reorganize curricula (Lenburg, 1999).

After all the discussion, the question of why resources should be used to share what is currently being done still remains, especially if there are no obvious concerns and issues.

REASONS FOR REDESIGNING PROGRAMS, CURRICULA, OR COURSES

Collaboration among educators, employers, health care providers, and other stakeholders is an essential first step to meeting the needs of the changing education and workplace landscapes. Coonan (2008) addresses issues that demand change in nursing education. New graduates are not prepared for practice. A culture of continuous improvement, based on innovations in technologies, teaching/learning strategies, and the recognition of learners as active participants is needed.

Continued competence of nurses and other health professionals is not required after initial licensure or is assumed, based on completion of various educational programs. Patient and consumer competence to manage their health and prevent illnesses is not assessed by measurable outcomes. Public policy initiatives internationally, nationally, and at state levels are beginning to address the public's interest in having assurance that they receive competent, quality care (Jordan, Thomas, Evans, & Green, 2008).

Educational programs for nurses, health professionals, patients, and consumers may not stay current with new knowledge, standards, and regulations. Traditional programs focus on content from textbooks, articles, commercial education materials, and other sources which may not be current. There is no ability, time, and resources available to continually update curricula and content. Nursing students purchase specialty texts that are very lengthy. Patient-education materials may be used for long periods of time. Materials used for consumer education may not address key areas such as literacy levels and the needs of multicultural and diverse populations.

Changes in regulations, standards, best practices, and new evidence all contribute to the need for revised educational offerings. The continual revision of educational programs, based solely on updating content, is impossible to manage and does not address learner outcomes that demonstrate the achievement of competence.

To overcome some of these barriers to implementing CBE in postsecondary education, there needs to be a holistic view. Graduates must be prepared to meet current needs of society, but also have the essential skills required to maintain and heighten their competence to meet future needs. There are examples of institutions and organizations that have successfully implemented competency-based programs.

Examples of CBE

1. Western Governors University was created as a CBE institution. Students demonstrate competence rather than completing discrete courses for a degree, and have multiple pathways to demonstrate competence. Initial assessments indicate what students know and can do, related to required competencies. The processes for determining competencies and assessments are based on input from external stakeholders, content experts, and experts in assessment and measurement (Western Governors University [WGO], 2008).
2. Maricopa Community College District has an educational model with competencies linked to specific curricula. The development process starts on the campus level in order to have input from internal and external stakeholders, including individuals with different types of expertise: content experts, instructional designers, and information technology specialists (Maricopa Community College District [MCCD], 2008).

3. Maricopa Advanced Technology Education Center (MATEC) is a division of Maricopa Community Colleges. "MATEC's primary educational products are instructional modules that are tailored to the goals of the National Science Foundation (NSF) Advanced Technology Education program. MATEC modules blend key elements of core curriculum (e.g., physics, math, and chemistry) from secondary and postsecondary programs with specific knowledge/skills that technicians need in the high-tech industries. This integrated curriculum enables students to further refine their general knowledge while acquiring industry-relevant abilities that prepare them for a desirable career" (MATEC, 2008 at http://matec.org/cd/cd.shtml).

4. MATEC curriculum development and instructional design is based on standards of quality education and training, principles of educational psychology, and established methods of job-skills training. Competency-based instruction was selected because it uses an appropriate instructional platform that is effective for both education and job training (MATEC, 2008 at http://matec.-org/cd/cd.shtml).

5. The Learning and Assessment Center at Michigan State University (2008) includes all the practice disciplines. The mission is to assess whether students are proficient in key tasks and support curriculum changes that are competency driven.

CBE has many elements that fit with the goals of nursing education programs. Nursing leaders have promoted this approach since the early 1900s.

Competency-Based Nursing and Health-Related Education Programs

Competency in both nursing education and practice is widely discussed today because the gap between the two areas continues to widen at all levels of educational preparation (Tilley, 2008). The concept of competency in nursing education in the United States was addressed in the early 1900s as state legislatures passed laws to regulate the practice of nursing by establishing education requirements and licensure. By the 1970s, state boards of nursing also started regulating competency after licensure (Whittaker, Smolenski, & Carson, 2000).

Carrie B. Lenburg has been a leader in the development of competency-based nursing education since the 1970s. The increasing complexities of health care and recognition by consumers, professionals, and regulators support the need for prelicensure nursing education programs and RNs' need to demonstrate competency (Lenburg, 1999). The Competency Outcomes and Performance Assessment (COPA) Model provides a comprehensive framework for integrating essential concepts required to develop and implement competency outcomes, learner center activities, and reliable, valid assessment methods (Lenburg,1999).

Coonan (2008) addresses the need for educational innovations to insure that new graduates have the knowledge and skill set to function in complex health care environments. This requires use of evidence for educational improvements, new programs, and new methodologies. The following are examples of competency-based programs:

1. Alverno College (2008) is an international leader in nursing education. The programs focus on preparing graduates to demonstrate outcomes and abilities required to effectively practice nursing. The college has a tradition in liberal arts and provides integrative, experiential, and reflective methods to nursing education. Assessment is viewed as an essential component of student learning.

2. Acute care environments are becoming more complex, and a frequent challenge is assuring there is sufficient competent nursing staff. Hospitals are responsible for competency assessments which are ongoing. A comprehensive program includes initial development, knowledge and skills maintenance, consultation for educational needs, and remedial activities. Performance Based Development Systems (PBDS) support the use of a variety of assessments methods and options for managing the required documentation (Whelan, 2006).

3. Davidson (2008) completed an online survey of health education and health promotion professionals to determine the job relevance of the National Commission for Health Education Credentialing (NCHEC) competencies, as well as preferred training formats. The respondents identified 4 out of the 35 competencies as being most needed for their jobs, and 5 competencies for which they needed additional training. Their preferred methods for continuing education were attending the American College

Health Association annual meeting and completing home self-study print materials. The results of this study are useful for planning educational offerings that focus on the needs of the health education professionals to maintain their competence.

4. There are multiple lists of public health nursing competencies. Cross et al. (2006) could not find a valid instrument to measure any changes in public health nursing competency that occurred over time. An instrument was developed to reflect 195 public health nursing activities. The authors went through multiple stages of development and had a panel of nursing experts validate the data. This project demonstrates how a group of nurses found a way to actually use assessment of competencies in practice settings.

5. Pharmacology education is responding to external forces, such as legislative and accrediting bodies, who are asking for better accountability. The mandate is that programs determine what graduates are able to do (*outcomes*) and provide evidence that they have demonstrated these abilities (*assessment*). The article is one in a series that describe the processes for developing competency-based pharmacology programs. This article focused on the detailed processes for developing assessment. Following these guidelines will prepare graduates for their new responsibilities (Anderson, Moore, Anaya, & Bird, 2005).

6. Leadership in maternal and child health (MCH) requires a wide variety of skills that go beyond clinical or academic disciplines. Leaders in all settings must respond to rapidly changing health environments. An MCH conference in 2004 created a framework for developing future MCH leaders. The purpose was to determine leadership skills that cut across areas, identify training needs, and select methods to assess leadership competencies. The leadership competencies are forward-thinking. They include the concept of "capability," adapting to new situations, and producing new knowledge. An innovative aspect is "capstone" projects to assess competencies. The MCH nursing group believes the approach can be used as a model in diverse health, education, and social service settings. The group not only identified essential competencies and methods to assess them, but also provided a model for other disciplines (Mouradian & Huebner, 2007).

The examples of CBE programs, described in the previous section, were adopted to update and/or improve the programs. In other instances, CBE is selected because of specific issues or concerns.

Examples of Implementation of Competency-Based Nursing and Health-Related Education Programs, Based on Identified Needs

The following examples demonstrate different approaches to implementing competency-based programs, based on identified needs:

■ The World Health Organization (2007) is recognized for its efforts on many fronts to improve the health of all people. Strategic Directions were developed for 2002–2008 and included five key intervention areas to improve nursing and midwifery services:
  ○ Health and Human Resources Planning
  ○ Management of Health Personnel
  ○ Practice and Health Systems Improvement
  ○ Education of Nurses and Midwives
  ○ Leadership and Governance

■ Specific guidelines for implementing the strategic directions for strengthening nursing and midwifery services in the African region were developed for 2007–2017.

   The goal is to make the strategies explicit and also consider the needs of individual countries. The education guidelines addressed the need for regulatory bodies and professional associations to:

1. Develop country-specific nursing and midwifery education and service standards for nursing and midwifery practice.
2. Define essential or core competencies for nursing and midwifery practice in relation to scope of practice and practice standards as stipulated in the national regulatory framework.
3. Promote development of a competency-based approach to curricula design for nursing and midwifery education programmes (World Health Organization Regional Office for Africa, 2007).
4. The Australian Nursing and Midwifery Council (ANMC) (2005) first adopted national standards for registered nurses

in the early 1990s. By 2004–2005, the ANMC wanted to make sure the standards were current for practice and met regulatory requirements. The standards are broad and serve as a framework for assessing competency. The four domains are: professional practice, critical thinking and analysis, provision and coordination of care, and collaborative and therapeutic practice. Methods for assessing competency include self, peers, recipients of care, and supervisors. The process is completed annually and required for license renewal.

5. The National Health Service, in the United Kingdom, recognized the need for nursing graduates to be "fit for practice and fit for purpose." Prior to 2000, the educational model was based on apprenticeship principles. The new model retained existing positive practices. New recommendations included more interprofessional collaboration and learning, as well as having the standards, required for registration, based on outcome competencies (Fordham, 2005).

6. The University of Colorado School of Nursing celebrated its centennial in 1997–1998 and reflected on all the contributions it had made to nursing education in the state, nationally, and internationally. It was time to look to the future. Employer focus groups identified deficiencies in preparation of the graduates. The graduates themselves did not feel they had the entry-level competencies required for practice. The faculty determined principles on which to base curricular revisions that would retain the core values of the school. The curriculum would be:

   ● Competency based and outcome focused; modular and flexible.
   ● Accessible to learners who desired a degree or lifelong learning opportunities, and learner centered.
   ● Focused on the "real world" of evidence-based practice.
   ● Technology based (Redman, Lenburg, & Hinton-Walker, 1999).

7. The Oregon Consortium for Nursing Education (OCNE) was established in 2001 to respond to the acute nursing

shortage in that state. It is a partnership of community colleges and public and private university schools of nursing. The goal is to help schools of nursing increase their enrollments. Features of the consortium are:

- A shared curriculum taught on all the campuses.
- Students can complete an AAS degree at a local community college.
- Students can complete distance coursework for the bachelor of science degree in nursing without leaving their home communities.
- The curriculum is based on a set of core competencies.
- Shared use of resources such as simulation laboratories.
- Technology links for teaching/learning and communication.
- Agreements for shared student services.
- Agreements for shared academic policies.
- Shared purchasing of equipment and services.

8. The state of Texas has a model of differentiated entry-level competencies to identify the continuum of preparation from the licensed vocational nurse to doctorally prepared registered nurses. The document was developed with broad input from education, regulatory, and consumer groups. The identified competencies cover the spectrum of educational levels, and each builds upon the previous levels. The competencies consist of the knowledge, judgment, skills, and professional values expected of a novice nurse at graduation. The purpose of the document is to add precision and uniformity to educational outcomes. Nursing programs can use it to improve programs and support articulation for educational mobility ("Differentiated Entry Level Competencies," 2000).

9. The Nursing Emergency Preparedness Education Coalition (NEPEC) was founded in 2001 to assure there is a competent nurse workforce to respond to mass casualty incidents (MCI). "As part of the international community's overall plan for emergency preparedness in mass casualty incidents (MCI), nurses worldwide must have a minimum

level of knowledge and skill to appropriately respond to an MCI, including chemical, biologic, radiologic, nuclear, and explosive (CBRNE) events. Not all nurses can or should be prepared as First Responders. Every nurse, however, must have sufficient knowledge and skill to recognize the potential for an MCI, identify when such an event may have occurred, know how to protect oneself, know how to provide immediate care for those individuals involved, recognize their own role and limitations, and know where to seek additional information and resources. Nurses also must have sufficient knowledge to know when their own health and welfare may be in jeopardy and have a duty to protect both themselves and others (NEPEC, 2001).

10. The NEPEC consists of organizational representatives of schools of nursing, nursing accrediting bodies, nursing specialty organizations and governmental agencies interested in promoting mass casualty education for nurses. The NEPEC facilitates the development of policies related to MCIs as they impact nursing practice, education, research, and regulation. There are several focus areas for the organization. One is identifying MCI competencies for nurses in academic and practice settings.

11. The MCI competencies were developed in three stages: a review of existing competencies from other groups and organizations; responses to drafts of competencies; and a validation panel to provide feedback which the committee used to finalize the competencies.

A curriculum-based tool for medical and nurse educators has been developed. Ways were needed to collect, organize, and present resources for single or multidisciplinary groups of learners. The open source Moodle (Modular Object-Oriented Dynamic Learning Environment) Learning Management System was used for competency mapping (CMI) and to create a curriculum-building interface (CBI). The CMI provides a way to take high-level competencies, divide them into logical subunits, and attach specific learning objectives, activities, and assessments such that individual learning activities and assessments can support teaching multiple competencies. The CMI has keyword codes and searchable collections of learning activities and assessments organized by competency. It is possible to collect and download educational resources stored in Moodle. Faculty can build custom curricula and track student progress toward achieving competency. This open source Moodle module is suitable for all types and levels of professional education programs (Voss, Jackson, Goodkovsky, Chen, & Jerome-D'Emilia, n.d.). This is an example of addressing the need to organize and manage essential information in CBE programs. Institutions, programs, and courses have adopted CBE approaches to meeting the changing internal and external expectations to assure learners are competent at the end of their educational endeavors.

Although there is interest and efforts to address competency-based nursing and related health education have begun, there are areas that need consideration before such programs are accepted and implemented:

1. Agreement on common terms, definitions, meaning, and expectations.
2. Validation of methods and approaches to measure competencies.
3. Collaboration among all parties; the public, nurse educators, providers, professional associations, and regulators (Jordan, Thomas, Evans, & Green, 2008).

It is possible to begin to change attitudes and beliefs about CBE. Voorhees (2001) provides a checklist of good practices, based on research done by the National Postsecondary Education Cooperative (NPEC). Changes need to start at the institutional/organizational levels. The principal aspects are:

1. Senior leadership members are open to change and become the advocates for change.
2. Competency-based activities are included in the institutional/ organizational culture.
3. Competency assessments are directly linked to goals and learning experiences.
4. A diverse group of stakeholders participate in determining the competencies.
5. Faculty and staff participate in making decisions about assessment instruments and processes.

6. All types of assessment processes and instruments are carefully evaluated for reliability, validity, credibility, and cost.
7. Competencies are specifically defined so they can be appropriately assessed.
8. Multiple competency assessments provide the data essential for policy and outcome decisions.
9. Critical decisions for improving student learning outcomes are derived from assessment data. Assessment results are collected for individuals and aggregated for meaningful reporting.
10. Institutions/organizations promote experimentation and innovation.

Institutional/organizational support for competency-based initiatives, at all levels and all types of nursing education programs, helps get the processes started. The need for change is based on many factors. New internal and external expectations, concerns about the effectiveness of current educational outcomes, and changes in health care environments are driving forces. Schools of nursing, professional groups, regulators, and employers have taken on the challenge of redesigning teaching and learning in their environments.

The future of competency-based learning for nurses may have these features:

1. A common model for all nurses in all roles.
2. Regulatory initiatives should be pilot tested.
3. The use of technology and evidence as a basis for nursing actions.
4. Global approaches to assuring safety and quality of care for individuals, groups, communities, and society as a whole (Jordan, Thomas, Evans, & Green, 2008).

Nursing education programs have the shared responsibility, with all other interested parties, to prepare graduates who are competent to begin their practice in complex health care environments. This can be accomplished through authentic partnerships between nursing education and external stakeholders.

SUMMARY

CBE addresses the need to have graduates of nursing and health-related programs prepared for entry-level positions in their practice areas. Educators, employers, students, consumers, and external stakeholders all can contribute to making this a reality. Having a clear understanding of CBE is the first step in making the decision to implement CBE. The implementation of CBE requires a change in philosophy. Essential competencies, based on current standards and evidence, are established. Developing valid and reliable assessments to demonstrate what graduates know and can do is the key to assure competence.

CHAPTER 1 ACTIVITY

You have completed reading chapter 1 and now need to consider how CBE will improve learner outcomes in your institution or organization. Use Exhibit 1.1 to identify ways to implement CBE.

Exhibit 1.1

List issues/concerns related to learner outcomes in your current educational programs or courses.

Identify issues/concerns in your organization or institution.

Seek input from coworkers, colleagues, students, and other stakeholders; do they have similar and/or different concerns/ issues?

Determine the current status of the issues/ concerns; what is the status and what would you like the learner outcomes to be? Review Tables 1.1 and 1.2 for examples.

Match your needs to CBE; how can CBE be used to improve your outcomes?

REFERENCES

Alverno College. (n.d.). *Ability based curriculum.* Retrieved September 20, 2008, from *http://www.alverno.edu*

Anderson, H. M., Moore, D. L., Anaya, G., & Bird, E. (2005). Student learning outcomes assessment: A component of program assessment. *American Journal of Pharmaceutical Education, 69*(2), 256–268.

Australian Nursing and Midwifery Council. (2005). *National competency standards for the registered nurse.* Retrieved October 15, 2008, from http://www.anmc.org.au/docs

Bradshaw, A. (1997). Defining "competency" in nursing (Part I): A policy review. *Journal of Clinical Nursing, 6,* 347–354.

Bradshaw, A. (1998). Defining "competency" in nursing (Part II): An analytic review. *Journal of Clinical Nursing, 7,* 103–112.

Citizen Advocacy Center. (2006). *Implementing continuing competency requirements for health care professionals.* Retrieved September 20, 2008, from www.cacenter.org/cac/continuing_competence_requirements

Coonan, P. R. (2008). Educational innovation: Nursing's leadership challenge. *Nursing Economic$, 26*(2), 117–121. Retrieved September 15, 2007, from http://www.euro.who.int/document/e86582.pdf

Cross, S., Block, D., Josten, L. V., Recklinger, D., Olson-Keller, L., Strohschein, S., et al. (2006). Development of the public health nursing competency instrument. *Public Health Nursing, 23*(2), 108–114.

Davidson, E. S. (2008). Perceived continuing education needs and job relevance of health education competencies among health education and promotion practitioners in college health settings. *Journal of American College Health, 57*(2), 197–209.

Dearing, R. (1997). *Higher education in the learning society.* London: Report of the National Committee. Retrieved September 15, 2008, from www.ex.ac.uk/dearing.html

del Bruno, D. (2005). A crisis on critical thinking. *Nursing Education Perspectives, 26*(5), 278–282.

Differentiated Entry Level Competencies of Graduates of Texas Nursing Programs. (2000). *Texas Board of Nurse Examiners.* Retrieved September 15, 2008, from *www.bne.state.tx*

Eraut, M. (1998). Concepts of competence. *Journal of Interprofessional Care, 12*(2), 127–139.

Evers, F. T., Rush, J. C., & Berdrow, I. (1998). *The bases of competence: Skills for lifelong learning and employability.* San Francisco: Jossey Bass.

Faris, R. (1995). *Major reforms in training systems in three countries.* Victoria, BC, Canada: Ministry of Skills, Training, & Labour. Retrieved October 15, 2008, from www.members.shaw.ca/rfaris/docs/1995Nations.pdf

Fordham, A. J. (2005). Using a competency based approach to nursing education. *Nursing Standard, 19*(31), 41–48. Retrieved September 1, 2008, from http://futurehealth.ucsf.edu/pdf_files/recreate.pdf

Girot, E. A. (1993). Assessment of competence in clinical practice: A phenomenological approach, *Journal of Advanced Nursing, 18,* 114–119.

Gonczi, A. (1994). Competency based assessment in the professions in Australia. *Assessment Education, 1*(1), 27–44.

Griener, A. C., & Knebel, E. (Eds.). (2003). *Committee on health professions education summit: A bridge to quality.* Washington, DC: National Academies Press.

Jordan, C. Thomas, M. B., Evans, M. L., & Green, A. (2008). Public policy on competency: How will nursing address this complex issue? *Journal of Continuing Education in Nursing, 39*(2), 86–91.

Juceviciene, P., & Lepaite, D. (2005). *Competence as derived from activity: The problem of their level correspondence.* Retrieved October 20, 2008, from http://www.education.ktu.lt/evaco/competence.html

Kerka, S. (1998). *Competency based education and training: Myths and realities.* Columbus, OH: Clearinghouse on Adult, Career, and Vocational Education (ACVE). Retrieved September 15, 2008, from www.cete.org

Learning and Assessment Center at Michigan State University. Retrieved September 20, 2008, from http://lac.msu./edu

Lenburg, C. B. (1999). The framework, concepts and methods of the competency outcomes and performance assessment (COPA) model. *Online Journal of Issues in Nursing, 4*(3). Retrieved September 15, 2008, from http://www.nursingworld.org/ojin

Maricopa Advanced Technology Education Center (MATEC). *History and foundation.* Retrieved October 15, 2008, from http://matec.org

Maricopa Community College District. (2008). Retrieved August 10, 2009, from http://www.maricopa.edu/workforce/curriculum.php

Mouradian, W. E., & Huebner, C. E. (2007). Future directions in leadership training of MCH professionals: Cross-Cutting MCH leadership competencies. *Maternal Child Health Journal, 11,* 211–218.

Nagelsmith, L. (1995). Competence: An evolving concept. *Journal of Continuing Education In Nursing, 26*(6), 245–248.

National Council of State Boards of Nursing. (2005). *Meeting the ongoing challenge of continued competence.* Chicago, IL: Author.

National Council of State Boards of Nursing. (2008). *NCLEX-RN pass rates.* Retrieved October 15, 2008, from https://www.ncsbn.org/Table_of_Pass_Rates_2008.pdf

Norman, I. J., Watson, R., Murrells, T., Calman, L., & Redfern, S. (2000). *Evaluation of the validity and reliability of methods to assess the competence to practice of pre-registration nursing and midwifery students in Scotland.* Final report to the National Board for Nursing, Midwifery and Health Visiting for Scotland.

Nursing Emergency Preparedness Education Coalition (NEPEC). Retrieved October 15, 2008, from http://www.nursing.vanderbilt.edu/incmce/competencies.html

Oregon Consortium for Nursing Education (OCNE). Retrieved October 15, 2008, from http://www.ocne.org

Pew Heath Professions Commission. (1998). *Recreating health professional practice for a new century: The fourth report of the Pew Health Professions Commission.* Retrieved September 20, 2008, from http://futurehealth.ucsf.edu/pdf_files/recreate.pdf

Redman, R. W., Lenburg, C. B., & Hinton-Walker, P. (1999). Competency assessment: Methods for development and evaluation in nursing education. *Online Journal of Issues in Nursing, 4*(3). Retrieved September 15, 2008, from http://www.nursingworld.org/ojin

Tilley, D. D. (2008). Competency in nursing: A concept analysis. *Journal of Continuing Education in Nursing, 39*(2), 58–64.

U.S. Department of Education. (2006.) A test of leadership: Charting the future of U.S. higher education. Washington, DC: Author.

Voorhees, R. A. (2001). *Measuring what matters: Competency-based learning models in higher education.* San Francisco: Jossey-Bass.

Voss, J. D., Jackson, J. M., Goodkovsky, V., Chen, Y., & Jerome-D'Emilia, B. (n.d.). *Mapping & distributing competency-based curricula: Tools and techniques.* Retrieved October 15, 2008, from http://www.iamse.org/conf/conf12/abstracts/Assessment/ed%20-%20jackson.htm

Watson, R., Stimpson, A., Topping, A., & Porock, D. (2002). Clinical competence assessment in nursing: Review of the literature. *Journal of Advanced Nursing, 39*(5), 421–431.

Wendt, A., & Marks, C. (2007). *An analysis of post entry-level registered nurse practice. CLEAR Exam Review.* Chicago, IL: National Council of State Boards of Nursing.

Western Governors University, About WGU. Retrieved September 20, 2008, from *https://www.wgu.edu*

Whelan, L. (2006). Competency assessment of nursing staff. *Orthopaedic Nursing, 25*(3), 198–202.

While, A. E. (1994). Competence versus performance; which is more important? *Journal of Advanced Nursing, 20,* 525–531.

Whittaker, S., Smolenski, M., & Carson, W. (2000). Assuring continued competence, policy questions and approaches: How should the profession respond? *Online Journal of Issues in Nursing.* Retrieved October 30, 2008, from http://www.nursingworld.org/ojin

World Health Organization Regional Office for Africa. (2007). *WHO Guidelines for implementing strategic directions for strengthening nursing and midwifery services in the African region, 2007–2017.* Brazzaville, Republic of Congo: Author.

Worth-Butler, M., Murphy, R. J. I., & Fraser, D. M. (1994). Towards an integral model of competence in midwifery. *Midwifery, 10,* 225–231.

Xu, Y., Xu, Z., & Zhang, J. (2001). A comparison of nursing education curriculum in China and the United States of America. *Journal of Nursing Education, 41*(7), 310–316.

ADDITIONAL RESOURCES

Internet Sites for Discipline-Specific Accreditation Standards

The following sites are examples of CBE standards for selected disciplines:

The American Association for Health Education (AAHE) addresses National Health Education Standards for achieving excellence in K-12 health education programs and for health education students who must exhibit competence in carrying out planned programs. *http://www.aahperd.org/aahe/pdf_files/standards.pdf*

The Commission on Dental Accreditation expects each school to develop specific competency definitions and assessment methods in the context of the broad scope of general dental practice and reflect an evidence-based definition of general dentistry. *http://www.ada.org/prof/ed/accred/standards/predoc.pdf*

The Council on Education for Public Health has a primary focus on educational outcomes, on the competencies, professional knowledge, and skills students acquire through their course of study. Overall program effectiveness relates directly to student achievement, and excellence in education is linked to proficiency in practice. *http://www.ceph.org/i4a/pages/index.cfm?pageid=n3274*

The Joint Commission on Accreditation of Healthcare Organizations (JCAHO) accredits all types of health care organizations. They are dedicated to helping health care organizations improve and sustain quality of care and patient safety that translates into practical strategies and real results. The burden is on employers to assure all their staff is competent to provide quality and safe care in all areas of an organization.

The Liaison Committee on Medical Education specifies that educational objectives include what students are expected to learn (knowledge, skills, behaviors, and attitudes) and relate to the competencies that the profession and the public expect of a physician. The associated outcome measures should assess whether and how well graduates are developing these competencies as a basis for the next stage of their training. *http://www.lcme.org/standard.htm*

The Magnet Recognition Program was developed by the American Nurses Credentialing Center (ANCC) to recognize health care organizations that provide nursing excellence. By recognizing quality patient care, nursing excellence, and innovations in professional nursing practice, the Magnet Recognition Program provides consumers with the ultimate benchmark to measure the quality of care that they can expect to receive.

The National Council for Accreditation of Teacher Education (NCATE) has a comprehensive quality assurance system for the teaching profession that recognizes there is a continuum for preparation that includes professional associations, state agencies, and K-12 education standards that are aligned to NCATE standards and have assessments to assure the public that teachers who graduate from NCATE-accredited institutions are well prepared to help their students learn. *http://www.ncate.org/public/ncatrole.asp?ch=1*

The National League for Nursing Accreditation Commission (NLNAC) accredits all levels of nursing programs. http://www.accrediting-comm-nlnac.org/

Internet Sites Related to CBE Initiatives and Standards

The following sites provide examples of CBE programs:

Education Resources Information Center (ERIC) is an online digital library of education research and information. ERIC is sponsored by the *Institute of Education Sciences* (IES) of the *U.S. Department of Education*. ERIC provides ready access to education literature to support the use of educational research and information to improve practice in learning, teaching, educational decision making, and research. *http://eric.ed.gov/ERICWebPortal/custom/portlets/recordDetails/*

Geneva Foundation for Medical Education and Research: Health Service Quality Improvement after Normal Delivery Competency-Based Training Package. *http:// www.gfmer.ch/Endo/PGC_network/Health_service_quality_im provement.htm*

Minnesota Department of Health Emergency Preparedness Training and Exercises The Healthcare Personnel Emergency Preparedness (HPEP) site outlines broad competencies, as well as subcompetencies, in emergency preparedness. *http:// www.health.state.mn.us/oep/training/*

National Center for Education Statistics "Defining and Assessing Learning: Exploring Competency-Based Initiatives." *http://nces.ed.gov/pubsearch/pubsinfo.asp? pubid=2002159*

North Central Regional Educational Laboratory "Outcome based" education: An overview. *http://www.ncrel.org/sdrs/areas/issues/envrnmnt/go/go4outcm.htm*

2 Developing and Applying Competency-Based Education

MARION G. ANEMA

OVERVIEW

This chapter begins with a focus on the essential elements of competency-based education (CBE) and answers the question, "Why should we have CBE programs?" There are different models that can be used to develop CBE courses or programs, based on the setting or needs. The Lenburg Model is used in this chapter to outline how to develop a CBE course or program.

There are a variety of ways to organize content, learning activities, and assessments, and the most common approaches are discussed. Courses and programs are also delivered in different modes, such as in a traditional classroom or via distance learning. A key part of CBE is using multiple assessments to measure competency; the rationale for this approach and types of assessments are described. It is also important to consider the range of learning styles.

Approaches to developing competencies are explained, along with guidelines related to reliability, validity, precision, and costs. The remainder of the chapter explains how to get started, how to develop a

CBE project, and describes project planning tools. Activities (found at the end of the chapter) provide the opportunity to develop a project plan.

INTRODUCTION

The commitment to initiate a CBE program is a major undertaking and requires support throughout the entire organization or institution. Chapter 1 included examples of CBE being adopted at institutional, program, and course levels. Obtaining a commitment to CBE at all levels provides many types of support: personnel, financial, and other resources. Those directly involved in developing a program or revising a curriculum need detailed knowledge of the processes, whereas others who facilitate the processes need specialized skills related to instructional design and psychometrics. Content experts also are essential to determining the required competencies and the appropriate assessments. It is important to recognize the essential elements of CBE.

ESSENTIAL ELEMENTS OF CBE

Hoppe (n.d.) asked the question, "Why should we do competency-based health professions education? Her answers are:

- CBE begins with the end in mind;
- The main focus is always on the outcome, rather than processes;
- Processes are important when the outcomes of the competencies are considered.

Hoppe (n.d.) goes on to explain how CBE is really different. Competencies are developed based on expectations of what graduates should be able to do. The assessments are specifically tied to the competencies. The results are used to adjust learner experiences and promote competency in specific areas. Program and course information is also reviewed to determine whether any changes are needed.

Traditional and competency-based programs have similar processes for development of programs and courses. Table 2.1 compares the differences in end results. In traditional programs, the end results are that learners either pass or fail a course. They move forward or complete

Table 2.1

COMPARISON OF TRADITIONAL AND COMPETENCY-BASED HEALTH EDUCATION END OF PROGRAM RESULTS

TRADITIONAL HEALTH EDUCATION PROGRAMS		COMPETENCY-BASED HEALTH EDUCATION PROGRAMS	
Pass the course	Progress in the program	Demonstrate competency	Progress in the program
Fail the course	Repeat the course OR exit the program	Does not demonstrate competency	Remediation: Learner responsible/ accountable; Faculty/mentor support
		Reassess	
		Demonstrate competency	Progress in the program

a program when they pass. If they fail, they may have the option of retaking the course or may not continue in an education program. Even when learners pass a course, they may not be competent in specific areas, but their overall grade or final score is acceptable. In CBE programs, learners demonstrate competence, based on assessment results, and move forward. If learners fail and do not demonstrate competence, they have remediation options. Learners are responsible for seeking additional learning resources. Learners have faculty or mentor support. There are options for reassessment and the learners can progress or complete programs.

Figures 2.1 and 2.2 illustrate the similarities between the traditional and CBE approaches.

The development of a CBE program or course requires a different frame of reference compared with traditional educational programs. In the classification of behavioral or learning outcome objectives, there are different levels to describe mastery of the skills, knowledge, and values that demonstrate competency. Learners may be at a knowledge or comprehension level where they can describe how to carry out a

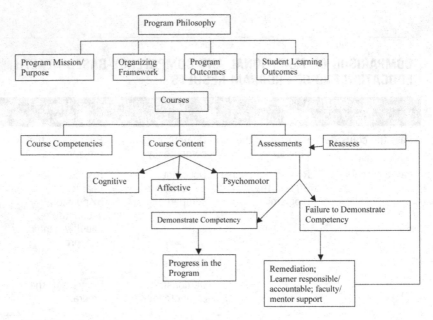

Figure 2.1 Competency-based health education programs.

procedure, explain the process for critical thinking, or identify the elements of collaboration in a work setting. The next level is to perform a skill, calculate a dosage, document information, or recognize the essential information related to a clinical problem. Learners who can apply what they know, analyze situations or information, integrate it into a clinical situation, assess the outcomes of their actions, and make changes as needed, are competent. At the beginning of practice, nurses may be competent and develop proficiency as they gain experience.

Differences are mainly in the areas of:

- Current educational processes that focus on the acquisition of knowledge and the ability to demonstrate that knowledge. Student-learning outcomes in CBE include the same areas but go further, and require that learners actually use the knowledge to carry out nursing activities. The nursing program at Alverno College uses an ability-based approach. It is expected that students do something with what they know. Students must be able to

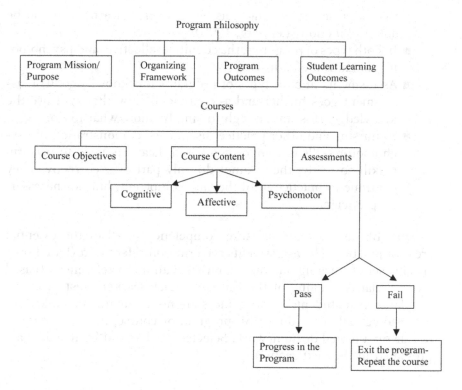

Figure 2.2 Traditional health education programs.

use what they know and know how to do by applying it competently and proficiently (Hoppe, n.d.).

■ CBE course objectives are carefully aligned to educational activities that support achievement of competency. Traditional programs usually have long lists of objectives that are content-focused. Learners are given a great deal of knowledge, and it is assumed they can apply it to specific situations.

■ CBE focuses on competency outcomes and uses verbs such as apply, demonstrate, integrate, and implement. Traditional course/unit objectives require students to list, discuss, describe, recognize, and recall.

■ CBE course content is based on needs of the practice community. Traditional programs keep adding content because it is "essential." This approach does not address competency, but assumes

that because "everything" has been covered, learners should be able to function (Lenburg, 1999).
- In both types of programs, the cognitive, affective, and psychomotor domains are addressed.
- Assessments in both types of programs test knowledge. CBE assessment goes further and asks students how they will use the knowledge. It is not enough to simply know what to do.
- In nursing and other practice disciplines, demonstration of psychomotor skills is competency-based. Learners need to perform a skill correctly; they cannot do only part of it correctly. They continue to practice until they are competent, but not necessarily proficient.

In CBE, assessments measure competency in all of the essential areas of practice. The assessments are criterion-referenced (based on a specific set of learning outcomes), rather than norm-referenced (based on the relative ranking of the learners). Each learner must meet the standards, and students' performances are not compared or ranked. In order to actually develop a CBE program or course, it is necessary to decide on a model or framework. Selected models and frameworks are presented in the next section.

MODELS OF CBE

A curriculum needs to reflect the mission and philosophy of the institution/organization. For CBE to be successful, everyone needs to understand what it is, have the resources and training needed to implement it, and have the processes in place for evaluation and improvement. Once those elements are in place, a model or framework is selected to provide a structure for a program or courses. The purpose is to determine the content and competencies.

Lenburg (1999) developed a Competency Outcomes and Performance Assessment (COPA) model. It is holistic and requires that practice-based outcomes are integrated. It is useful in both formal education and service environments. The model is simple but comprehensive, and asks four essential questions:

- What are the essential competencies and outcomes for current practice?

- What indictors define the competencies?
- What are the most effective ways to learn the competencies?
- What are the most effective ways to document that learners and/ or practitioners have achieved the required competencies?

These questions provide guidance for program and course development. Another perspective focuses directly on practice settings.

Wright (2005) developed a competency assessment model for health care practice settings. The main features are:

- A collaborative process between staff and managers is used to identify competencies;
- The competencies are prioritized according to need and reflect the continuing changes in workplaces;
- Verification of competencies is employee-centered;
- A variety of verification methods includes guided reflective practice approaches, outcome measurement of daily work activities, and methods to develop critical thinking skills;
- A culture of success is created by focusing on the organizational mission and promoting positive employee behaviors.

Another group, The Australian Primary Health Care Research Institute (2006), selected a framework for developers of CBE. They must:

- Clearly align objectives with workforce-related outcomes;
- Identify common learner outcomes in different health-related programs;
- Be responsive to the complexity of the environments that impact change;
- Actively manage the change processes.

The Nursing Council of New Zealand (2001) developed a competency-based framework to regulate professional nursing throughout the country. The goal was to have a common understanding of what nurses need to know and do. They designed a competency assurance framework that includes regulatory, health, and professional sectors in order to link all the requirements for initial and continuing registration of nurses. The framework builds on the existing evaluation and monitoring processes already in place for nursing education programs.

The Council considered CBE development a priority because:

- It would be done at a high level and link changes in practice and monitoring with regulatory requirements;
- The Nursing Council could promote professional growth to meet the changing needs of the health care environment;
- The Ministry of Health released a Medical Credentialing Framework and required a response from the Nursing Council.

To receive a competency-based practice certificate as a registered nurse, applicants must practice according to standards for registration and also meet 11 competency performance criteria. The competencies are:

- Communication
- Cultural Safety
- Professional Judgment
- Management of Nursing Care
- Management of the Environment
- Legal Responsibility
- Ethical Accountability
- Health Education
- Interprofessional Health Care
- Quality Improvement
- Professional Development

Another aspect of developing CBE programs and courses is determining how the content and assessments will be organized. The National League for Nursing Accrediting Commission (2006) described how the curriculum starts with the philosophy and mission, continues through an organizing framework to learner outcomes (competency statements), and to organizing content and assessments to achieve the desired outcomes.

ORGANIZING STRATEGIES

There is a variety of ways to organize content, learning activities, and assessments. In nursing and health-related programs, common traditional organizing strategies still used today are:

- Medical Model—organized by diseases and body systems, terminology, and specific skills;
- Simple-to-Complex—learning is organized in sequences, such as basic skills to more complex ones, or from individuals to groups to communities;
- Stages of Illness—health is presented first, followed by acute care nursing, rehabilitation, and chronic care nursing (Iwasiw, Goldenberg, & Andrusyszyn, 2005).

Two other organizing strategies are more commonly used today:

- Interdisciplinary—requires collaboration and team work between several disciplines. Planning, developing, and teaching are done jointly;
- Outcomes—requires that outcomes are determined first. Learners achieve competencies and the outcomes are evaluated (Iwasiw, Goldenberg, & Andrusyszyn, 2005). There are different ways to deliver educational programs, and making such decisions is part of the planning process.

Delivery Approaches

Today, there is a variety of approaches to presenting educational programs and courses. The philosophy and mission of an organization/institution determine the approaches to delivering educational programs. The type of content, availability of learning resources, learner characteristics, and cost are also factors in making the decision.

Face-to-face instruction is the most common approach. Learners are in one place, and a teacher or leader is responsible for ensuring the goals of each session are achieved. Technology such as videos, computer learning modules, and simulations can be used as teaching strategies. Independent distance learning takes place when students complete work on their own and turn it in. This is done electronically or by mail.

Distance education approaches are varied and depend on the degree and types of technology used. Learners may enter a Web-based classroom and complete assignments in that setting. It can be asynchronous (independent responses to questions and postings to others in the class) or synchronous (interaction with others in discussion and chat areas).

There can also be synchronous video and phone interactions. Combinations of teaching and learning strategies are often used to provide a variety of learning experiences and options. Multiple assessments are developed to measure the essential student learning outcomes that demonstrate achievement of competencies.

MULTIPLE TYPES OF ASSESSMENTS

Assessments are directly related to measuring the competencies. Determining which domains to assess is the first step. Domains include the identified competencies and learning statements. In professional programs, the domains and competencies are based on national standards as well as licensure and certification requirements. Assessments are organized and developed for specific purposes:

- In formal education programs, which have practice components, assessments measure cognitive, affective, and psychomotor competencies;
- Staff development programs include assessments that address competencies required for hiring, maintaining competence, and gaining competence in new areas of practice;
- Patient/consumer education usually focuses on specific health- and disease-related topics. Assessments may include psychomotor components if skills are needed. Cognitive areas include knowledge, comprehension, application, and evaluation. Changes in health behaviors are based on the affective domain (values, beliefs, attitudes, emotions) and are essential competencies.

Assessments can be objective- or performance-related:

- Objective assessments usually have predetermined, correct responses. Examples are multiple choice tests, oral responses to questions, and short-answer written responses. The focus is on what learners know and know how to do;
- Performance assessments focus on what learners can do with their knowledge. Higher level assessments of critical thinking, synthesis, affective domains, and psychomotor skills have a range

of responses. Examples are simulations, portfolios, essays, journals, and skills demonstrations.

Using multiple assessment approaches to assess learner attainment of competencies has advantages. Objective assessments can focus on knowledge, concepts, and basic skills. Assessments are often given at various levels, simple to complex, so learners demonstrate a foundation. For example, learners will need to have foundational competency in human body structures and functions in order to make clinical decisions related to providing care. Students, patients, and consumers need to demonstrate competence related to terminology and physiologic concepts related to a particular health issue. They can then advance their level of competency to critically analyze what they know, synthesize the information, and apply it to a situation. Adult learners have a variety of ways they learn.

LEARNING STYLES

Knowles (1970) focused on how adults learn differently from children. He collected information based on observations about best practices found in the literature, and what teachers find successful. Learning is an internal process. Learners control their own learning and teachers/mentors serve as facilitators. Knowles used the term *andragogy* as the art and science of helping adults. The characteristics of andragogy include:

- Adult learners assume responsibility for their learning and are self-directed;
- Use experiences and apply new knowledge to solve real problems;
- Collaboration is part of the learning process;
- Motivation is internal and driven by curiosity (Billings & Halstead, 2005).

Learners have different learning styles, and have the opportunity to demonstrate their competency in different ways.

APPROACHES TO DEMONSTRATING COMPETENCY

Creating multiple assessments requires matching a learning domain with an appropriate type of assessment. The delivery mode also determines what is possible. If the learners are in the same place, it is possible to include oral presentations, questioning, and group activities. Technology continues to advance, and synchronous approaches may also be possible. For example, live interactive classrooms at different locations allow students to interact.

It is easy to lecture and make presentations in front of a group and then measure learning outcomes. The most common assessment approaches are:

■ Paper/pencil or computer-based examinations;
■ Oral presentations with the teacher/mentor grading according to set rubrics;
■ Written assignments;
■ Demonstrations primarily for psychomotor skills.

The goals of CBE are to use a variety of approaches to measure competencies and recognizing differences in learners and delivery approaches. Additional approaches to determining competency include:

■ Integrating cognitive domain learning, such as critical analysis and synthesis;
■ Journaling that lets learners reflect and complete self-assessments. The affective domain is addressed;
■ Videotaping, which can measure psychomotor, cognitive, and affective domains, depending on the focus and complexity of a situation (Billings & Halstead, 2005).

The data collected from the different measures provide a holistic view of learner outcomes, including strengths and weaknesses. If the learner outcomes are very positive in some areas but much lower in other areas, there should be an evaluation of the different components. Additional information can be obtained from the learners and other experts to determine the problems and suggestions for improvement.

In a CBE approach, the competency assessments actually have to measure what is expected. They are developed using psychometric measurement principles. The cost of developing competencies is always a consideration.

RELIABILITY, VALIDITY, PRECISION, AND COSTS

Measurement principles include ensuring that the assessment methods are reliable and valid. Reliability means that assessments consistently measure the specified competencies. Validity refers to the level (high, moderate, or weak) that assessments measure what is expected (McDonald, 2002).

It is apparent that assessment measures must be precise. It is essential that the evaluations of assessments are consistent and done fairly. Different faculty, teachers, and mentors will review and grade assessments. Rationales for correct responses to objective assessments and sample grading notes are provided to the graders. Rubrics provide precision because they prove numerical values, based on precise descriptions. Table 2.2 provides examples of rubrics.

It takes a great deal of time to develop assessments. Faculty may be given time off from teaching responsibilities. Content experts may be hired to develop specific assessments. Publishers and educational companies have developed commercial products, and professional groups offer a variety of assessments related to their disciplines. When planning a change to CBE, cost is an essential element that must be addressed in the plan. How much will it cost? Another essential element is determining the format for reporting assessment results and actually using the data for improvement.

ASSESSMENT REPORTING AND USE OF RESULTS

Managing assessment data so the reporting is comprehensive and meaningful to the stakeholders is often overlooked when making early decisions about implementing CBE. Such decisions need attention at the beginning and throughout the planning processes. The benefit of changing how data is reported needs to be explained so stakeholders see the value of the change.

For example, if current ways of reporting are used for learner success, such as employing course grades, retention rates, degrees and certificates awarded, etc., competency of learners is not demonstrated, but is assumed. Everyone involved wants a clear presentation of the results of assessments and what additional work is needed for learners

Table 2.2

SAMPLE RUBRICS				
RUBRICS COMMON TO ALL	1 = NOT ACCEPTABLE	2 = REVISIONS NEEDED	3 = DEMONSTRATES COMPETENCY	4 = COMMENDABLE
Organization	Assignment does not follow required content and format areas	Assignment has missing format and content areas	Assignment contains all required format and content areas	Detailed inclusion of all format and content sections
Grammar, mechanics, punctuation	Major errors interfere with responses	Few errors interfere with clarity of responses	Few errors noted	Errors not detected
Citations and references in correct format	Contains major, repetitive errors	Contains a few major errors and/or many minor errors that distract from reading/ understanding content	Few errors detected	Errors not detected
Overall complete	Unacceptable	Needs revision	Meets competency	Exceeds expectations

to pass assessments. Additional sources for assessment reporting may include work experiences, portfolios, essays, journals, and samples of written artifacts such as manuscripts and PowerPoint® (PPT) slide presentations. The usual approach is that teachers calculate numerical grades that are converted to letter grades. Present systems are set up for that type of reporting and storing of data. New systems are required to store the large amounts of information CBE programs produce. Innovative systems can support ways to use and expand reporting options. Experts in these areas must be part of the development of CBE initiatives (Voorhees, 2001).

The major elements of CBE have been described. As the initial discussions about moving to CBE are in progress, it is useful to begin

Table 2.2 *(continued)*

SAMPLE RUBRICS

RUBRICS FOR SPECIFIC ASSIGNMENTS	1 = NOT ACCEPTABLE	2 = REVISIONS NEEDED	3 = DEMONSTRATES COMPETENCY	4 = COMMENDABLE
Cognitive				
Integrates a minimum of four adult learning principles into educational activities	No adult principles included	Only two adult learning principles included	Four adult learning principles included	More than four adult learning principles included
Affective				
Identify and examine positive and negative feelings when teaching individuals with mental illness	Does not include any feelings	Includes feelings but does not examine them	Includes feelings and examines them	Provides detailed account of feelings and their effects
Psychomotor				
Uses five indicated sterile techniques when preparing and self-administering an insulin injection	Does not use any sterile techniques	Omits two sterile techniques when self-administering insulin	Makes one minor error in sterile techniques when self-administering insulin	Demonstrates the use of all five sterile techniques when self-administering insulin

to develop a tentative plan. How is the project going to be accomplished, what is a reasonable timeline, what resources are needed, how will personnel be trained, and who has the expertise to work on the plan?

GETTING STARTED

Individuals or groups within an institution/organization may have learned about CBE and realize that what is currently being done needs to be improved or revised. They cannot just start making changes on their own. For example, educators may want to change a course they are teaching. Educators in a staff development or education department may want to revise all the courses. A health educator or nurse in a community setting may simply want to update selected programs. In any of these situations, there is the responsibility to develop a plan for the change and share it with the decision makers.

The plan may be informational only, because the changes will result in improvements based on data and not require additional resources. An example would be learners scoring low on part of a quiz and their satisfaction responses indicating any problem areas. The person responsible for the quality of the program can make changes based on the data. The process is repeated to measure quality. This could be a good opportunity to make program revisions based on CBE principles.

In most situations, a departmental committee or working group will work on changes and then follow the processes for approval. There may be only one additional approval or several levels. It is usual that approvals are needed at various levels.

An issue is how much time and effort should go into developing a comprehensive plan when it is not known whether there is any interest in, or the resources for, making a change. Voorhees (2001) pointed out that support from administration within an organization and from external stakeholders is essential. Discussing CBE at meetings and sharing information is one way to get started. Faculty, staff, administrative, and advisory meetings are venues to begin discussions. Use existing data and comments from others, including students, to identify what needs to improve. Once there is support and interest, a plan should be developed.

DEVELOPING A CBE PLAN

A plan may be very simple if the project is small, perhaps to change a patient education course, or complex if it involves several departments or entire organizations. If there is interest in preparing a grant application, the specific grant-writing guidelines are used. Grant applications have many of the same requirements that are included in a project plan. Determine what format is appropriate to develop the plan.

Stakeholders and other interested persons need to understand why CBE is an option for educational programs, the main processes, expected learner outcome competencies, and the resources required. It is important to include links to additional information. A project plan to use a CBE approach includes:

- Linking the program with the organization/institution mission, goals, and expected learner outcomes;
- Developing or using an existing educational model;
- Determining the internal and external stakeholders;
- Describing the context of the program within the organization/institution (culture, structure, and people);
- Identifying essential resources (personnel, space, learning aids, technology for program implementation and evaluation);
- Projecting the costs and benefits of a CBE approach (budget).

There are many other more detailed steps and decisions when undertaking a CBE project. Project planning is part of any organization. It can be very complex, such as building new facilities or determining how to improve learner outcomes for a single program or course. Consult with others in the institution/organization who have expertise in project planning. The project processes and format need to be consistent with established processes and guidelines. An institution/organization may have project planning tools in place.

PROJECT PLANNING TOOLS

Project planning systems and tools are available commercially or customized systems may be developed for specific uses. Everyone is very busy and may be at different locations and have different work hours. Scheduling face-to-face meetings is often very difficult. Phone conference calls are more flexible because participants can call from wherever they are, even in different time zones. Technology-based collaborative systems provide comprehensive options for planning projects. Features to look for in project planning tools, especially those that are technology based:

- Tools should be user friendly and set up for workspaces without users needing technical knowledge;

- Audio conferencing may be part of the planning system;
- Templates for charts are available to use for specific parts of the project;
- Documents and files are stored in different usable formats;
- Documents and files are kept in a single repository;
- Documents can be created and revised online;
- Charts, spreadsheets, formulas, etc., are available;
- Revisions to documents are tracked and all versions are available for review;
- Project tracking is part of the system;
- Files and documents are kept on a secure site;
- Collaboration teams are set up for the entire group and subgroups;
- The leaders encourage team members to actively participate.

Project planning needs to be comprehensive and have processes in place to assure the participants can effectively contribute and participate. A Gantt chart is an example of a system used to track the project.

Gantt Chart

A Gantt chart typically includes milestones, activities, responsible persons, and target dates for the different phases and completion of the entire project. Gantt charts are useful when scheduling and monitoring tasks are important. The chart also sets out the steps and time frames for each. It is a good communication tool because everyone involved can see what is happening.

The American Society for Quality provides resources, training, certification, and networking opportunities to professionals in health care. They have developed a model for project planning, a simple model that is useful for small projects:

- **Phase I: Initiation**—Determine scope of project: WHAT;
- **Phase II: Planning**—Determine tasks/activities of project: HOW;
- **Phase III: Execution**—Carry out the tasks/activities, monitor progress against plan, report progress, manage changes;
- **Phase IV: Completion**—Implement: stakeholders and users evaluate changes, collect and analyze data, and make improvements based on data.

A sample project plan is supplied at the end of the chapter in Exhibit 2.2. Links to examples of systems are also listed at the end of the chapter. Any project has to have persons designated to make sure the necessary steps are performed to achieve success.

DECISION-MAKING ROLES AND RESPONSIBILITIES

The organizational structure of an entity will have guidelines in place and processes for making decisions. In large, complex organizations, decision making may be done at department or unit levels. In smaller organizations, the staff and person in charge may jointly make decisions.

As mentioned earlier, all stakeholders need a voice in determining how CBE will be implemented. The starting point may be informational sessions to broad audiences so they understand CBE and why changes are being made.

SUPPORT FOR CBE

Support for CBE should start with both the internal and external stakeholders. Internal stakeholders are:

- Persons in administrative and managerial positions;
- Educators who teach courses;
- Staff persons who provide support services;
- Learners who participate in the program;
- Technology experts;
- Assessment and evaluation experts.

External stakeholders include:

- Governmental and public regulatory agencies;
- Accrediting organizations;
- Education and health-related associations;
- Researchers;
- Media services;
- Consumer groups.

It is evident that many different individuals and groups must have a voice in initiating a competency-based approach to education. Once a plan is developed, the information needs to be shared widely. An efficient way to share the information is with a summary.

SUMMARY OF A PLAN

Summaries may have the title of executive summary, abstract, project overview, project proposal summary, project analysis, or other similar names. The purpose of a summary is to provide leaders and decision makers with the essential information found in the project plan. It is assumed that the audiences who read a summary, may not read the entire plan or proposal. The summary is a stand alone document which allows the reader to review all the essential information and make decisions. Tips for writing a summary include:

- Organize the summary in the same format as the complete plan;
- Use only information that is in the plan, do not add anything new;
- The length varies, but may be very short (less than one page to much longer, 10 pages or more). A general guide is that the summary length be about 10% of the length of the plan. Short is better than long;
- The first sentence must capture the readers' interest;
- The main areas include issue or purpose, supporting evidence, cost/benefit analysis, and recommendations for action;
- It is important to include links to additional information.

Once there is interest and support for CBE and a plan is developed, it is time to keep moving the processes forward to gain approvals and begin the real work of implementing CBE. The next chapter describes the processes and issues related to implementing CBE in three different types of educational settings.

SUMMARY

A basic question about the benefits of CBE is answered. The focus is on the end results, preparing graduates who are competent to practice in their discipline. There are many decisions to make to start developing a CBE course or program:

- Selecting a model, based on the setting and needs of the learners;
- Determining how to organize content, learning activities, and assessments;
- How the course or program will be delivered;
- Including multiple assessments;
- Addressing statistical methods and processes.

The Lenburg Model is an example of how to develop a CBE course or program. An effective way to organize the development processes is to use a project plan. Following the steps in a project plan supports completing the various activities and tracking what is done and what still needs to be done. The following activities provide the opportunity to develop a project plan.

CHAPTER 2 ACTIVITIES

You have completed reading this chapter and now need to prepare a project plan. Use the list you compiled in Exhibit 1.1. Determine the focus and/or priorities for what you want to accomplish. What is feasible to actually complete in your organization or setting? Use the resources you already have: such as interested persons in your organization, support from other stakeholders, data from existing assessments, and research-based best practices. Use the sample plan as a guide to develop your own plan. Modify it to fit the type and complexity of the CBE course or program you want to develop. Use your completed plan to move forward with the CBE processes. The next chapter provides information about changing existing courses or programs. Applications to specific types of programs (formal education, staff development, and patient education) are included.

In chapter 1, the activities focused on making decisions about adopting CBE in your setting. The activities required for chapter 2 move the process forward by making critical decisions about specific elements of CBE for your program or course. After reading chapter 2 and reviewing the additional resources, do the following:

Exhibit 2.1

AREA	SET–NO	PRO	CON	DECISION
Organizational Mission	🔒			
Organizational Philosophy	🔒			
Framework/ Model				
Philosophy of Education				
Organizing Strategies				
Delivery Approaches				
Multiple Assessments				
Learning Styles				
Demonstrating Competency				
Reliability, Validity, Precision, Costs				
Assessment Reporting and Use of Data				
Developing a CBE Plan				
Project Planning Tools				
Decision Making Rolls and Responsibilities				
Support for CBE				
Plan Summary				

Exhibit 2.2

SAMPLE PROJECT PLAN

Project: Revise an 8-week Adult Diabetic Education Program from traditional to competency-based

Note: Highlight each task as it is completed.

Start and Finish Dates:

SEQUENCE	TASKS	KEY MILESTONES	TIME REQUIRED	COMPLETED WORK/ PRODUCT
Phase I 1/09-3/09	Initial discussions by interested staff	Group is committed to moving forward	2–3 months	
	Gather need and background information	Information collected		
	Prepare information sheet	Information sheet developed	2–3 months	
Phase II 3/09-6/09	Meet with internal administrator to gain initial support	Administrator offers support		
	Expand group to include additional stakeholders (community advocates, faculty, patients, professional groups, etc.)	Convene meeting		
Phase III 6/09-9/09	Explain CBE to group	Subgroup assignments are made	2–3 months	
	Develop subwork groups			
	Resources needed			
	Training required			
	Determine needs of learners			
	Review current course to determine what can be used for CBE			
	Specify how project fits within overall institutional planning processes			

(continued)

Exhibit 2.2 *(continued)*

SEQUENCE	TASKS	KEY MILESTONES	TIME REQUIRED	COMPLETED WORK/ PRODUCT
Phase IV 9/09-1/10	**Work focuses on determining:**	**Subgroup assignments are made (depending on expertise):**	5–6 months	
	Essential competencies	Educators		
	Content	Content specialists		
	Learning resources			
	Most effective ways to learn competencies	Course designers		
	Best ways to assess learning	Potential participants in course		
	Methods to document achievement	Psychometic experts		
	Develop evaluation processes for course			
	Determine training needs of educators and learners			
Phase V 1/10-3/10	Implement CBE course on a pilot group	Use multiple methods to measure student learning and outcomes	3–4 months	
	Collect outcome data	Time to complete course		
		Number who completed course		
		Level of achievement in each area		
		Survey, focus group, etc. to elicit positive/ negative comments from faculty, students, and support staff		

Exhibit 2.2 _(continued)_

SEQUENCE	TASKS	KEY MILESTONES	TIME REQUIRED	COMPLETED WORK/ PRODUCT
Phase VI 3/10-6/10	Decide how to use data for program improvement	Compare data from old course with new course	3–4 months	
		Make improvements based on data		
		Determine methods and time frame for reviewing data		
		Select methods and processes for reporting and sharing data		
		Consider presenting and publishing experiences in developing a CBE course and outcomes		

Set up a planning form to summarize your ideas and options (see Exhibits 2.1 and 2.2). Use the form to capture your ideas, share them with stakeholders, and track activities. The form can be developed as an Excel® spreadsheet. There are usually set items that will not change when transitioning to CBE. In Exhibit 2.1, the organization's mission and philosophy would not change, so a lock symbol can show that on the form. If available, create a Website workspace for everyone to access the documents, make changes, and share comments about revisions.

REFERENCES

American Society for Quality. (n.d.). _American Society for Quality—Knowledge center._ Retrieved October 30, 2008, from http://results/index.html?page=category&category=Measurement

Australian Primary Health Care Research Institute. (2006) Retrieved November 4, 2008, from http://www.acerh.edu.au/publications/Glasgow_APHCRI-Report_Sep06.pdf

Billings, D. M., & Halstead, J. A. (2005). *Teaching in nursing: A guide for faculty.* St. Louis, MO: Elsevier Saunders.

Glasgow, N., Wells, R., Butler, J., Gear, A., Lyons, S., & Rubiano, D. (2006). *Using competency-based education to equip the primary health care workforce to manage chronic disease.* Australian Primary Health Care Research Institute. Retrieved October 30, 2008, from www.anu.edu.au/aphcri

Hoppe, R. B. (n.d.). *Competency-based health professions education: Why should we do it?* Retrieved October 15, 2008, from http://lac.msu.edu/

Iwasiw, C., Goldenberg, D., & Andrusyszyn, M. A. (2005). *Curriculum development in nursing education.* Sudbury, MA: Jones and Bartlett.

Knowles, M. (1970). *The modern practice of adult education.* New York: Associated Press.

Lenburg, C. B. (1999). The framework, concepts, and methods of the competency outcomes and performance assessment (COPA) model. *Online Journal of Issues in Nursing, 4*(3). Retrieved October 30, 2008, from http://www.nursingworld.org/ojin

McDonald, M. E. (2002). *Systematic assessment of learning outcomes: Developing multiple-choice exams.* Sudbury, MA: Jones & Bartlett.

National League for Nursing Accrediting Commission (NLNAC). (2006). *Accreditation manual with interpretive guidelines for post secondary and higher degree programs in nursing.* New York: Author.

Nursing Council of New Zealand. (2001). *Towards a competency assurance framework for nursing.* Wellington, New Zealand: Author.

Voorhees, R. A. (Ed.). (2001). *Measuring what matters: Competency-based learning models in higher education.* San Francisco: Jossey-Bass.

Wright, D. (2005). *The ultimate guide to competency assessment in health care.* Minneapolis, MN: Creative Health Care Management, Inc.

ADDITIONAL RESOURCES

Central Desktop: Social Technology Platform for Business Collaboration Software for Teams, Departments & Enterprises. *http://www.centraldesktop.com/*

Project KickStart Pro 5 to generate ideas, solve problems, and increase efficiency. Useful for starting projects by asking the right questions to create new projects. *http://www.projectkickstart.com/products/project_kickstart.cfm*

Overview: Executive Summaries. *http://writing.colostate.edu/guides/documents/execsum/*

Standard Summaries. *http://writing.colostate.edu/guides/documents/standsum/*

Writing the Executive Summary of the Business Plan: How to Write an Executive Summary That Gets Your Business Plan Read. *http://sbinfocanada.about.com/od/businessplans/a/execsummary.htm*

3

Applying a Model to Develop and Implement a Competency-Based Education Program/Course

MARION G. ANEMA

OVERVIEW

This chapter provides an overview of the processes essential to implementing a competency-based education (CBE) program. Lenburg's (1999) Competency, Outcomes, and Performance Assessment (COPA) model requires an analysis of an environment where educational programs are offered. The model is grounded in principles of adult education, active and interactive learning, and demonstration of competency at the end of an instructional course or program. The model serves as a guide to examine and respond to four essential questions:

1. What are the essential competencies and outcomes for contemporary practice?
2. What are the indicators that define those competencies?
3. What are the most effective ways to learn those competencies?
4. What are the most effective ways to document that learners and/or practitioners have achieved the required competencies? (Lenburg, 1999).

The four questions are applied to three scenarios which address different types of educational offerings: academic, staff development, and client/consumer. Because of the emphasis on self-management, the client/consumer scenario considers the individuals with diabetes to be the educators. They have to educate themselves. For each scenario, an example is included from each type of educational setting. The activity provides a blueprint for answering the four questions in your own educational setting.

INTRODUCTION

Lenburg's (1999) COPA model provides a framework for determining content and competencies in instructional settings. Decisions are made by examining current health care environments and practice settings. Embedded in this approach is a commitment to adult learning principles, student-centered and interactive learning, practice-based outcomes, and multiple assessments of competencies.

COPA MODEL FRAMEWORK

The COPA model framework is straightforward and requires everyone involved in instructional development or revision to answer the following questions.

Question 1. What are the essential competencies and outcomes for contemporary practice?

The essential competencies must be determined and worded as specific competencies for the identified practice setting. Traditional objectives are often knowledge-based, rather than addressing how to use the knowledge.

Many individuals and groups have participated in determining competencies essential for practice. Regulatory organizations and agencies, professional groups, employers, and others concerned with the preparation of health care providers have developed regulations, standards, and guidelines. Based on all the previous efforts, Lenburg (1999) identified eight core practice competencies and the specific skill areas required. The core competencies are:

1. Assessment and intervention skills;
2. Communication skills;
3. Critical thinking skills;
4. Human caring and relationship skills;
5. Management skills;
6. Leadership skills;
7. Teaching skills;
8. Knowledge integration skills.

See Table 3.1 for the core practice competency list with subskills.

The framework is useful because the classification of competencies can be used in many different practice settings and in a variety of health-related professions. The list is a guide for the development or revision of a curriculum. It provides a focus for determining essential content for a program or course. Selection of essential content is made more difficult, even overwhelming, because of the amount of information available today. The framework can be used along with the expectations of internal and external stakeholders. Program accreditation standards state what content should be included in programs. Accrediting bodies for organizations and agencies include expected outcomes. Licensing boards and credentialing organizations specify requirements. The challenge is to use this information and develop outcome competency statements which indicate practice skills rather than knowledge.

Developers of courses and programs often understand how traditional objectives are stated. They may have previously developed programs and/or are familiar with them from their prior educational experiences. The key to shifting from "how to learn" to selecting content is to focus on practice outcomes.

Adkins (2004) describes how educational taxonomies developed by Bloom, Krathwohl, and collaborators have been used for decades as frameworks for instructional objectives, curriculum design, and assessments of achievement. Originally, they identified three overlapping human learning domains: cognitive, psychomotor, and affective learning. The three domains represent the knowledge, skills, and beliefs of a human performer (Adkins, 2004).

Outcomes are organized in taxonomies, which are systems used to categorize and classify things. A taxonomy, which is widely accepted for planning and evaluation purposes in instructional settings, has three areas: cognitive, affective, and psychomotor domains. Within

Table 3.1

CORE PRACTICE COMPETENCIES WITH SUBSKILLS

CORE COMPETENCIES	SUBSKILLS
Assessment and intervention skills	Safety and protection Assessment and monitoring Therapeutic treatments and procedures
Communication skills	
■ Oral skills	Talking and listening with individuals Interviewing and history taking Group discussion and interacting
■ Writing skills	Clinical reports, care plans, documentation of care Agency reports, forms, memos, and communicating through technology Articles and manuals
■ Computing skills (using technology, information processing, information management)	Related to clients, agencies, and other stakeholders Related to information search and inquiry Related to professional responsibilities
Critical thinking skills	Evaluation, integrating pertinent data from multiple sources Problem solving, diagnostic reasoning, creating solutions Scientific inquiry, research process related to evidence and best practices
Human caring and relationship skills	Morality, ethics, and legality Cultural respect, cooperative interpersonal relationships Client advocacy
Management skills	Administration, organization, and coordination Planning, delegation, and supervision of others Human and material resource use Accountability and responsibility, performance appraisal and QI
Leadership skills	Collaboration, assertiveness and risk taking Creativity and vision to formulate alternatives Planning, anticipating, and supporting with evidence Professional accountability, role behaviors and appearance
Teaching skills	Individuals and groups, clients, coworkers, consumers, and others Health promotion and health restoration
Knowledge integration skills	Nursing, health care, and related disciplines Liberal arts, natural and social sciences, and related disciplines

Adapted from Lenburg (1999).

each domain, the objectives are divided into levels. The leveling requires learners to master the lower levels before advancing to higher levels (Bastable, 2003). These three domains are addressed in all practice-based disciplines.

The levels in each domain go from simple to complex. For example, in the cognitive domain, a person needs some knowledge before applying it to a clinical situation. The levels of behavior for each of the domains demonstrate why it is easier to write objectives which focus on the lower levels.

The cognitive domain includes knowledge, comprehension, application, analysis, synthesis, and evaluation:

- *Knowledge* requires the learner to recognize or recall information;
- *Comprehension* requires the learner to define or summarize information;
- *Application* requires the learner to use ideas and principles in situations;
- *Analysis* requires learners to structure relationships between different types of information;
- *Synthesis* requires the learner to put parts together and create something new;
- *Evaluation* requires the learner to determine the value of something and critique it, using research, best practices, guidelines, and standards (Bastable, 2003).

The affective domain includes receiving, responding, valuing, organization, and characterization:

- *Receiving* requires the learner to be aware of an idea or fact and pay attention to what is presented;
- *Responding* requires the learner to be aware of an idea or situation, consider accepting it, and feel positive about a new experience;
- *Valuing* requires the learner to accept a theory or idea, accept the value of it, and be willing to continue to further accept its value;
- *Organization* requires the learner to organize, classify, prioritize, and integrate new values into an existing set of values;
- *Characterization* requires the learner to integrate new values into a total philosophical or world system and generalize them to diverse experiences (Bastable, 2003).

The psychomotor domain includes perception, set, guided response, mechanism, complex overt response, adaptation, and origination:

■ *Perception* requires the learner to be aware of sensations that are part of a task to be performed and includes reading directions and observing associated processes;

■ *Set* requires the learner to be ready to follow directions by verbal expressions or body signals;

■ *Guided response* requires the learner to imitate actions, with demonstration and coaching from an instructor;

■ *Mechanism* requires the learner to repeatedly perform the required steps in a task and blend the different steps into a set of expected actions for the entire task;

■ *Complex* overt response requires the learner to consistently perform a motor task independently with skill;

■ *Adaptation* requires a learner to modify or change a motor task based on individual or situational needs;

■ *Origination* requires the learner to create new motor tasks, based on previous knowledge and skills (Bastable, 2003).

It has been suggested that the scope of the three domains is too limited for current times and should be expanded. Dettmer (2006) suggested the following expansion of the learning domains and introduces a new, fourth domain:

■ Cognitive domain adds "ideational functions of imagination and creativity";

■ Affective domain adds "internalization, wonder, and risk taking";

■ Psychomotor domain adds the "sensorimotor domain, incorporating five senses along with balance, spatial relationships, movement, and other physical activity";

■ A new, fourth domain referred to as "social" is introduced. This new domain addresses the "sociocultural processes that accompany thinking, feeling, and sensing/movement."

The revised domains can be used when the new terms precisely define the learning domains.

When the subdomains are examined, there are differences in what learners are required to do. Learners need to start at the lower domain levels to gain a foundation for higher level expectations. The lower-level domains are useful for formative assessment. Learners need to demonstrate they have the knowledge to move to the next levels. For example, knowledge, comprehension, receiving, responding, perception, and set are preparatory to action.

Traditionally, educators have focused on the lower levels: sharing facts, information, theories, and concepts. Educators are the focus of the teaching/learning experience because they give information to the learners. Assessments ask learners to demonstrate their knowledge and comprehension of a topic.

Faculty need to develop very specific indicators which include the behaviors (actions, responses) that are required for nursing practice. Critical elements are developed for each skill with the indicators that demonstrate competence. For example, the skill of communicating with a client who does not understand English would include actions such as using written materials, pictures, or including an interpreter. The focus is on actions that would support effective communication.

It is challenging to construct assessments at the higher levels. Assessments have to go beyond examinations and written assignments where learners can demonstrate their knowledge and comprehension of a topic. What will they do with the information they have? In the higher domain levels, learners are required to actively demonstrate their ability to use what they have learned. CBE focuses on the end product, and summative assessment is used to determine achievement of a specific competency. Formative evaluation is done along the way to determine whether learners are making progress. What will graduates be able to do that aligns with current practice standards? As the graduates enter practice they will change how they use their knowledge and skills to create new ways of practicing. Because CBE requires assessing learner actions, it is necessary to use action verbs to develop learning outcome objectives.

The key to developing practice outcome objectives is to select action verbs. Table 3.2 provides some examples. Developers need to focus on the desired practice outcomes when writing new objectives or revising existing ones. Chapter 4 explains in detail the processes for making

Table 3.2

COMPARISON OF TRADITIONAL AND COMPETENCY-BASED OUTCOME VERBS

TRADITIONAL VERBS	COMMENT	COMPETENCY-BASED VERBS	COMMENT
Define Apply Explain Memorize Recognize Identify State Know	The verbs in the first column could have several interpretations. They do not require the learner to do anything with the knowledge and skills presented in the instructional setting. These types of verbs typically assess examinations and written assignments.	Apply Demonstrate Choose Design Diagnose Plan Respond	The verbs in the third column are specific and require the learner to do something with the knowledge and skills presented in the instructional setting. These types of verbs assess the learner's doing something in practice and completing a product (patient-education materials, new forms to document care, presentation of a program, or using specific cues when interacting with clients).

Adapted from Bastable (2003).

those changes. The next step is to decide which indicators illustrate practice competencies.

Question 2. What are the indicators that define these competencies?

Behavioral objectives are intended to be guides to selecting learning activities, developing instructional materials, and designing methods. Objectives also help learners organize what they need to study. Learners know how to focus their time and efforts to achieve the objectives. An essential purpose of objectives is to serve as the basis for assessment or evaluation (Bastable, 2003).

Behavioral objectives are supposed to establish what learners are able to do. Currently, the majority of behavioral objectives in instructional settings do not relate to essential behaviors. Having learners define, memorize, explain, or recall does not result in observable behaviors.

The indicators must be specific and include only the behaviors that are required for demonstrating competence in a specific area. Critical elements address all the core competencies and must be specific for each skill or subsets of a skill. A set of critical elements contains single, distinct behaviors that can be observed. They are not steps in a process, but relate a competency to a particular ability (Lenburg, 1999). After the indicators are selected, educators must make decisions and select the best approaches and methods to help learners become competent.

Question 3. What are the most effective ways to learn the competencies?

To answer this question, everyone involved in the teaching/learning process needs to have a new perspective. Teachers in all types of instructional settings need to move from dispensing information to facilitating learning. This is done by engaging learners in the educational process. Rather than lecture being the main teaching approach, learning is achieved by interactions and collaborations.

For over 100 years, many college classes have been conducted in large auditoriums, with lecture as the main teaching approach. Over the next decades, research supported a shift from lecture to smaller groups so students could participate (Weimer, 2002). This shift has not been widely accepted, as nurse educators continue to use lecture as a primary method of instruction. There is concern that students will not get all the required content. For example, nursing clinical texts often have 1,500 pages. The amount of content in health-related programs expands daily. An issue with focusing on content is that students may remember a great deal, but do not understand the meaning and how it relates to other concepts. Adult learning principles support using prior life experiences and goals to gain knowledge. Obviously, learners need a foundation of knowledge to actually gain the competencies to practice. The value of CBE is that all levels of learning are addressed, but the main goal is to assess competency at the end of a learning experience.

Educators have a wide array of choices when selecting learning activities. They range from low to high technology. For example, cooperative learning can be carried out in traditional and distance settings. Discussions, group projects, peer tutoring, learning cells, and teams are examples of active learning that can be used in different learning environments.

Problem-based learning was used at Harvard Medical School in the 19th century and instituted at McMaster University Medical School in 1969. Supporters, such as John Dewey and Jerry Bruner, contributed to the philosophical development of the concept. The case method has been used in business and law programs and now is an accepted part of many other disciplines. Students must actively participate in solving problems related to workplace situations (McKeachie & Svinicki, 2006). Additional active learning strategies are games, simulations, portfolios, discussions, presentations, projects, and journaling (Lenburg, 1999). Using a variety of interactive methods supports learners' ability to become independent and empower them to be responsible for their own learning.

Question 4. What are the most effective ways to document whether learners and/or practitioners have achieved the required competencies?

The main undertaking is to develop performance assessments that are:

- Learner-centered and are at the highest level of achievement required by the end of a unit;
- Clear, specific, and concise so both the teacher and learner understand what is expected;
- Measurable and based on psychometric principles;
- Criterion-referenced, judged against predetermined standards;
- Summative, with measured outcomes at the end of a learning unit;
- Diverse, with support for multiple measures to determine competency (Lenburg, 1999);
- Consistent with practice setting or new behavior expectations for learners who completed a program or course;

■ Congruent with the other competencies expected by the end of a program (Lenburg, 1999).

The entire process of developing competency performance assessments requires careful attention to using the identified competency domains and subskills. The competencies are based on input from stakeholders, current professional standards, and regulatory requirements. The outcome statements consider all the activities and focus on the end product. Newly developed statements and revisions of existing objectives must meet the criteria described above. The assessment data are reviewed and revised as needed.

It is not possible to go though all the CBE processes without understanding them. When everyone involved participates in training and completes practice activities, there can be collaboration and clarification. The continuing work will go smoothly. It is helpful to have someone who is knowledgeable about CBE who can serve as a resource person.

There are benefits for everyone who participates in CBE. Learners use their prior knowledge and experience as a foundation for new learning. Individually, learners can move through the processes at different rates. They do not have to wait for others to reach milestones. Teachers have data to support instructional outcomes and know that students have the knowledge and skills to do what is expected of them at the end of a program or course. Employers and the public have confidence that graduates are competent to practice in their disciplines. Three examples using the COPA model are described next. The examples focus on programs in academic, staff development, and patient/consumer settings.

Faculty need to develop very specific indicators that include the behaviors (actions, responses) that are required for professional practice or maintaining health. Critical elements are developed for each skill with the indicators that demonstrate competence. The focus is on actions that would support effective communication. The four COPA questions are presented in the next sections.

The development of a systematic and comprehensive plan for assessment is based on psychometric principles. Each competency is examined to determine what type of assessment will effectively demonstrate competency. This is the most complex aspect of transitioning to a CBE approach. Chapter 4 describes the processes in detail and provides specific steps for developing competency outcome statements. A training session is needed before the CBE process begins. Resources necessary for making these decisions include accreditation licensing and professional standards, evidence and best practices, and input from employers.

APPLICATION TO ACADEMIC EDUCATION PROGRAMS

Setting: The School of Nursing is part of a public university with 15,000 students. It is located in a metropolitan area and has a diverse student body of 900 Bachelor of Science in Nursing (BSN) students. Six hundred students are prenursing, and 300 are taking 5 semesters of nursing courses. There are 50 nursing faculty who teach in teams, based on their specialty areas. They recently received recommendations from the state board of nursing and their nursing accreditation organization. The information and data include the following:

- One hundred and fifty prenursing students apply each year for admission to the program, and 30 do not meet the admission requirements, mainly in the areas of an overall low grade-point average and grades of D in the science courses (a minimum grade of C is required);
- One hundred and twenty are admitted, and 30 students do not pass the first clinical nursing course (25% fail). They are allowed to repeat it once. Ten students who pass the first course decide nursing is not for them or drop for personal reasons. Eighty students move forward in the program;
- There is about a 3% attrition rate during the second, third, and fourth semesters due to failures and personal issues;
- Approximately 74 students (61.7%) graduate each year;
- The pass rate on the NCLEX-RN examination for licensure just meets the minimum required by the state board of nursing. The pass rate has been declining for the last three years, from 85% to the current 78%. If it goes any lower, the program may not continue to be approved;
- Sixty graduates become licensed the first time they take the NCLEX-RN examination and 14 do not. When the 14 graduates retake the examination, on the average, 50% will not pass;
- Employers realize that both attrition and inability of graduates to become licensed contribute to the continuing nursing shortage in the area;

- Faculty are concerned about all the resources that are expended for the program with unsettling results;
- The students who do not graduate and the graduates who do not become licensed face uncertain futures in their personal and professional lives.

The faculty meet to analyze the information and realize changes need to be made in the teaching/learning processes to improve outcomes. Based on the data, the faculty discuss further how they are teaching and how students are learning. They identify the following areas:

- Teaching focuses on covering massive amounts of content;
- Students pass courses but miss many critical areas;
- Students complain about doing the same patient care plans over and over throughout the program;
- Attrition because of failures and personal reasons is greater than desired;
- The pass rate on the NCLEX-RN licensing examination barely meets board of nursing and national standards;
- Employers identify that the graduates have limited critical thinking and integration skills.

The faculty hope they can make selected changes which will decrease attrition in all the nursing courses and improve NCLEX-RN pass rates. Part of their reasoning is that they need to show improvements in the outcomes, especially the NCLEX-RN pass rate for the next graduating class. They review Lenburg's (1999) COPA model to see how to apply it to this situation.

The faculty meet to analyze the current information and realize changes need to be made in the teaching/learning processes to improve outcomes. They organize their ideas under the COPA model.

Question 1. What are the essential competencies and outcomes for contemporary practice?

The areas of changes are focused on decreasing attrition in the nursing courses and increasing the NCLEX-RN pass rate in the next graduating class. To begin, the faculty perform the following actions:

■ Conduct a review of current standards, research, best practices, and expectations of new graduates to practice competently;
■ Invite the nursing program external advisory group, selected faculty representing all the courses, and a few students from each class to meet and provide input;
■ Each course leader meets with his/her team to look at the current course objectives to determine whether they focus on practice.

Result: The competencies are arranged under the eight core competencies identified by Lenburg (1999).

Question 2. What are the indicators that define the competencies?

Faculty select the competencies that are congruent with their courses. For example, the beginning courses require the acquisition of psychomotor skills. Each clinical course has a section related to cultural competence, and the advanced courses have an emphasis on critical thinking in case management. They compare current objectives with the newly identified competencies and make plans to revise existing ones.

Result: For each unit in a course, one third of the objectives will be revised to relate to practice competencies. Each unit will also include one activity to engage students in learning.

Question 3. What are the most effective ways to learn the competencies?

Faculty currently present the majority of the content by lecture. With changes in some of the objectives, they discuss how to change the course assignments to actively focus on practice. Different approaches are discussed for performance assessments and may include case studies, group projects, and the development of standard clinical care plans and presentations. Additionally, objective assessments will include scenarios that require making clinical decisions.

Result: Each team will select appropriate, practice-focused assessments, based on the revised objectives and indicators.

Question 4. What are the most effective ways to document that learners and/or practitioners have achieved the required competencies?

A process for evaluating any changes in student outcomes is developed. The items focus on attrition and the NCLEX-RN pass rate. Because instruments and data are available for other measures, additional data will continue to be collected for student and employer satisfaction. Additionally, qualitative data will be collected related to faculty reflections on the changes. An open-ended questionnaire is developed for faculty reflections. Benchmarks (desired outcomes) are determined for each of the measures (see Table 3.3). Faculty believe that completely revising all the courses is the ideal, but given the short time frame, this is a start.

Result: Data are collected after each semester and compared with the previous semester. It is especially important to review the first set of data after the change. Are there improvements in the measures? If not, what additional revisions are indicated? There needs to be attention to continuous improvement so attrition decreases and the NCLEX-RN pass rate increases.

Example of an Application in an Academic Setting

Faculty and staff at Northwest Missouri State University chose multiple measures to directly assess certain competencies. They used the Academic Profile to assess writing skills, college-level reading, and critical thinking of undergraduates. However, they also developed their own assessment instrument whereby students were asked to read multiple documents about a real issue or problem and then state their positions or justify the best solution to a problem in writing. Faculty designed this approach to determine whether students were mastering the necessary writing competencies. The writing faculty worked together to develop and implement scoring rubrics to assess student work. Undergraduates were required to take this writing assessment at the end of their second writing course. Students were typically given a series of short, related readings (often from newspapers or magazines) about a controversial topic and then asked to respond to specific prompts. (National Center for Education Statistics 2002; *http://nces.ed.gov/pubs2002/2002159.pdf*)

Table 3.3

BENCHMARKS FOR ACADEMIC PROGRAM OUTCOMES

AREAS OF EVALUATION	CURRENT OUTCOMES	BENCHMARKS (DESIRED OUTCOMES)
Attrition	Total attrition is 38.7%	The attrition rate will decrease by 10% in the first year after the changes and another 10% in the second year. Attrition in the 2nd, 3rd, and 4th semesters will decrease by 1% in the first year after the changes and another 1% in the second year.
NCLEX-RN pass rate	Pass rate is 78%	The pass rate will increase to 85% in the first year of changes and 5% increase each year after that, and be maintained at a minimum of 95%.
Course grades	Students who earn grades of D or F fail a course.	The number of D and F grades will decrease in proportion to the number of students who pass a course.
	Less than 10% of students earn an A in clinical courses.	Moving to a competency-based approach will increase the number of A's by 3% each year until it is maintained at 15–20%.
Student satisfaction	The current surveys indicate that 60% of students have overall satisfaction scores of <3 on a 5-point scale.	Student satisfaction scores will increase by 10% each year until 90% is reached and maintained.
Employer satisfaction	The current surveys indicate that 50% of employers have overall satisfaction scores of <3 on a 5-point scale.	Employer satisfaction scores will increase by 10% each year until 90% is reached and maintained.
Faculty reflects on changes and relates them to moving to a competency-based approach.	There is no current data because this is new information.	Faculty will be able to identify and relate positive outcomes to a CBE approach.

The next section presents a staff-development example. Competency assessment is adapted to each environment. The assessment processes can be positive or negative, depending on how they are designed, implemented, and evaluated.

APPLICATION TO STAFF-DEVELOPMENT PROGRAMS

Setting: Valley Medical Center is located in the Midwestern town of Valley Springs. It serves the immediate community of 50,000 and the surrounding areas with a population of 100,000. The medical center has 200 inpatient beds, emergency, medical, surgical, obstetric, and outpatient units, diagnostic and surgical centers, and four primary care satellite clinics. Martha Johnson is an experienced administrator and was hired six months ago as the vice-president of nursing and patient services. The previous nurse administrator had worked at the medical center for 10 years before she retired. The medical center is service and community oriented. It offers a variety of programs. Ms. Johnson has found the environment to be positive and the staff committed to the patients and communities they serve.

A major project is to prepare for the next Joint Commission (formerly JCAHO) accreditation visit due in one year. Measuring and verifying the competency of staff is a major focus. The current system is based on performance elements determined by administrators and managers. Both internal and external standards are interpreted to develop a performance program. Ms. Johnson would like to have a CBE system in place because she knows it will meet the Joint Commission standards, is congruent with the medical center's goal to be recognized for the quality of care provided, and nurses, from novice to expert, can continue to develop their competence.

Performance evaluation has its roots in Frederick Taylor's time and motion studies and Henry Ford's application to the assembly line, where performance was specified down to the smallest detail. Saul Sells developed a model for initial screening of prospective pilots, based on criteria, and then assessing their performance in combat (Steltzer, 2003).

Performance evaluation evolved into a system to determine compensation. It was believed that salary adjustments, either an increase or a decrease, would drive employee performance. The only way to get an increase was to perform at least at an acceptable level or higher, if possible. Employees who performed at a substandard level might have their compensation decreased (Steltzer, 2003).

A major issue with such a system was lack of clear statements or objectives to describe the different levels of performance. In addition, using such an approach has little to do with the recruitment and retention of competent workers. Other elements, such as job satisfaction, a positive work environment, and opportunities for personal and professional development are essential.

Mager (1975), a noted educator, developed a system for criterion-referenced instruction (CRI). The system focused on the knowledge and skills (competencies) needed to successfully perform a job. The CRI is suited to all levels of nursing practice because health care environments are dynamic and require continuous learning and adaptation.

Currently, performance appraisal systems focus on a developmental process. Employees have opportunities to develop the required skills, as well as advance within the organization by continually improving what they are able to do. Effective performance appraisal systems have the following characteristics:

- Individual job objectives are aligned with organizational goals;
- Employees know and understand the organization's performance expectations;
- Employees receive feedback about job performance;
- Employee strengths and weaknesses are identified;
- A collaborative approach is used to develop an improvement plan (Clark, 2009).

Ms. Johnson reviews information from the previous JCAHO report and becomes aware of a concern about catheter-associated urinary tract infections. Valley Medical Center had a high rate and was cited for that issue. Infection prevention and control are a high priority because more and more organisms are multidrug resistant (MDROs). "In 2008, the Center for Medicare and Medicaid Services (CMS) began to cease reimbursement for selected infections should they occur during a hospital stay" (Soule, 2009).

Patients who are especially vulnerable to infection are those with severe disease and have compromised host defenses from underlying medical conditions, such as recent surgery or indwelling medical devices like urinary catheters and endotracheal tubes (Siegel, Rhinehart, Jackson, & Chiarello, 2006). Based on the information, Ms. Johnson meets with the staff-development department members to discuss the need for a program to assure staff are competent in preventing hospital-acquired infections, especially those related to indwelling urinary catheters. The COPA model provides the framework for developing the program.

Question 1. What are the essential competencies and outcomes for contemporary practice?

"Infection prevention is among the highest priority issues for the Joint Commission and Joint Commission Resources for 2009. There is worldwide interest in and concern about a number of issues among patients, consumers, the media, regulators and others" (Soule, 2009).

"The Joint Commission has added the issue of MDROs to the National Patient Safety Goal (NPSG) as .07.03.01. NPSG .07.03.01 directs hospitals and critical-access hospitals to implement evidence-based practices to prevent health care-associated infections (HCAI) due to MDROs, and provides a phase-in period for getting systems in place by 2010" (Soule, 2009).

The essential competencies for this health care issue are to reduce MDROs associated with indwelling urinary catheter infections. The outcomes include the Lenburg core practice competencies:

- Assessment and intervention skills to monitor and formulate preventive measures related to infections;
- Communication skills to share reports and new information, and present educational programs;
- Critical thinking skills to evaluate strategies for prevention;
- Human caring and relationship skills to formulate strategies to prevent infections and promote collaboration;
- Management skills to organize prevention and monitoring activities;
- Leadership skills to formulate and create new interventions to achieve goals;
- Knowledge Integration skills to critique and synthesize information from diverse sources.

Question 2. What are the indicators that define the competencies?

The education program developed will need to be comprehensive and involve all employees. The type and amount of training will be directly related to their roles and responsibilities in the medical center. The educational program will include a number of indicators.

At the end of the educational program the staff will be able to:

- Implement administrative system changes to ensure prompt and effective communication about the status of the problem, new initiatives, and continued education;
- Provide the necessary number and appropriate placement of hand-washing sinks and hand-rub dispensers containing alcohol in the facility;
- Maintain staffing levels appropriate to the intensity of care required;
- Enforce adherence to recommended infection-control practices;
- Directly observe and provide feedback to staff on adherence to recommended precautions;
- Develop a "How-To Guide" for implementing change;
- Analyze the organization structure, process, and outcomes when designing interventions;
- Design global and unit/department-specific practice-related interventions;
- Intensify the frequency of MDRO educational programs for health care personnel, especially those who work in areas in which MDRO rates are not decreasing. Provide individual or unit-specific feedback when needed;
- Apply information from the Campaign to Reduce Antimicrobial Resistance in Healthcare Settings to reducing MDROs (Siegel, Rhinehart, Jackson, & Chiarello, 2006; *www.cdc.gov/drugresis tance/healthcare/default.htm*)

Question 3. What are the most effective ways of learning competencies?

Valley Medical Center employees have a wide range of educational backgrounds, expertise, and responsibilities. An educational program

Table 3.4

STRATEGIES AND EXAMPLES FOR LEARNING COMPETENCIES

LEARNING OUTCOMES	WAYS TO LEARN COMPETENCIES	EXAMPLES OF LEARNING ACTIVITIES
Communication system	Learning how to navigate the Website can include: Explicit directions; Individual and small group sessions; Self-directed tutorial; Refresher sessions to address specific problems.	Administrative support messages. Rationale for systemwide changes required with "How To" guide. Video clips and narrative for specific content. Space for Q's and A's and staff suggestions.
Appropriate equipment is in place	Develop a list of equipment and supplies recommended. Assign staff to determine whether it is appropriate.	Specific lists would be developed for areas such as patient care units, environmental services, laboratory, X-ray, food service, etc.
Adequate staffing levels	Administrators, managers, and monitoring team review current staffing levels and compare them with recommended standards.	A plan to meet staffing recommendations is developed as part of the system strategic plan and includes innovative strategies to increase efficiency, implement comprehensive screening, clustering high-risk patients, and rapid sharing of data.
Enforce adherence to standards	Organize a monitoring team with a representative from each service/department. The team will review all data and information and propose benchmarks for success. They will select methods for monitoring progress toward goals.	A comprehensive approach to collect, review, and use data is essential. Actively involving staff can change behavior and develop a culture of change. A standard reporting format is used to keep everyone informed of progress and problem areas.
Directly observe staff	Monitor assigned to directly observe staff.	Staff-development team will design rubrics and guides for specific tasks.
Analyze organization structures and processes	Administrators, managers, and monitoring team will determine what structures and processes are in place which support the initiative or impede it. Cross-training of staff may be needed, new equipment and supplies may be needed, and current procedures may need to be revised.	

(continued)

Table 3.4 (continued)

STRATEGIES AND EXAMPLES FOR LEARNING COMPETENCIES

LEARNING OUTCOMES	WAYS TO LEARN COMPETENCIES	EXAMPLES OF LEARNING ACTIVITIES
Design practice interventions	Multiple ways to learn can include self-instruction using an online video and narrative, printed materials, group discussions at the unit or department level, small-group or individual practice sessions, return demonstration with feedback, and collaboration/participation in improvement activities.	Video with a narrative on the Website, PowerPoint® presentations, individual CDs, short handouts that highlight new information and progress, review of information at unit/departmental meetings, one-on-one practice, demonstration, and feedback.
Increase educational efforts in selected areas	Review of data and explanation of the meaning by knowledgeable persons.	Develop protocols to address problems that continue. Have specific intervention to address specific problems; if infection rates do not drop using the standard approaches, then the next level could include additional observation and laboratory cultures. All options should be included at some level to control the problem.
Apply information from the "Campaign to Reduce Antimicrobial Resistance in Healthcare Settings" to the problem.	A list of resources will be on the system Website to support individual responsibility for learning. Staff members will be directed to check out new information.	Condense new information and focus on application to the problem. Share and discuss new information at unit/departmental meetings. Post short reminders in unit/department areas.

to reduce MDROs associated with indwelling urinary catheter infections will address the needs of all the learners. A comprehensive program must be adopted throughout the facility and should target the unit or area. Because so much of the data will be from laboratory reports, this information must be shared in formats that can be easily understood by everyone in the organization. A template for interpreting, summarizing, organizing, and presenting the data is essential. Changing behavior is a key to reducing the problem. The medical center culture must support these efforts (Siegel, Rhinehart, Jackson, & Chiarello, 2006).

Setting up or revising an existing process is a major undertaking in any organization. There are many more detailed steps and processes than presented. The purpose is to provide examples of the types of competencies needed, throughout an entire organization, to have everyone competent to address the problem. Table 3.4 identifies ways to learn the competencies and some examples.

The last step in the COPA model addresses creating competency-based examinations and assessments.

Question 4. What are the most effective ways to document that learners and/or practitioners have achieved the required competencies?

Health care organizations must meet many internal and external standards for all aspects of the hospital or other entity. Wright (2005) explains that the same questions in the COPA model are used in her outcome model. She adds that leaders need to create a culture of success which focuses on the organization mission, as well as encouraging positive employee behaviors. Organizations evolve and change to meet new demands in health care environments. Employees need help and support to grow professionally and move forward in the same direction as the organization. When recruiting, hiring, and retaining employees, there should be a good fit between the organization and what it values and the employee's professional values and goals.

Documentation of the congruence, with the expected outcomes, should have multiple verification options. For this initiative, several of them suggested by Wright (2005) are suitable:

- Return demonstrations;
- Self-assessment;
- Peer review;
- Discussion/reflection groups;
- Mock events/surveys;
- Quality improvement monitors.

As the learning activities are developed, appropriate assessments are determined. Adult learning principles, different ways of learning, selecting information to be learned, roles/responsibilities of learners, organizational goals, and the availability of technology all contribute to the need for multiple assessment.

It is also important to understand the stage of competency expected at the time of hiring, during initial employment, and once experienced on the job. The expected outcomes are developed for the initiative to decrease MDROs, with a focus on urinary tract infections. It is essential to develop competencies that are attainable. In this example, the competencies selected are the first priority for Valley Medical Center. The organization will continue to work on the other required assessments, but put time, effort, and resources into the priority.

According to Wright (2005), the role of managers is to work with employees to determine whether they have completed the required competencies, based on the verification methods. Elements of documentation include:

- Verification of completion of all required competencies;
- Determination of the level of competence based on the rubrics (unsatisfactory, satisfactory, competent, etc.);
- Action plan to address specific areas, related to expected outcomes;
- Identify how managers will support the employee and the organization mission.

The Valley Medical Center staff will all need to become competent in their areas of expertise to reduce the problem. Staff development is not just formal classes and checklists. In this scenario, the opportunities to work on developing parts of the initiative, contributing to the decisions, reviewing data, and learning new competencies promote active learning strategies.

Example of an Application in a Staff-Development Setting

The Certified Health Education Specialists (CHES) examination is a competency-based tool used to measure possession, application, and interpretation of knowledge in the Areas of Responsibility for health educators delineated in *A Competency-Based Framework for Health Educators* (2006). Consisting of 150 multiple-choice questions, the CHES examination is offered in paper-and-pencil format at college campuses throughout the United States. Although there are approximately 120 testing sites currently registered, any campus with a testing service is eligible to become a testing site.

Basis for the CHES Examination.   The CHES exam is based on Areas of Responsibility, Competencies, and Subcompetencies that were reverified by the findings of the National Health Educator Competencies Update Project (CUP), a 6-year multiphased national study of a representative sample of 4,030 self-identified health educators. The 163 validated Subcompetencies aligned with 35 Competencies and 7 Areas of Responsibility were first incorporated into a revised CHES examination in October 2007.

The third scenario addresses CBE programs for patients and consumers. The National Commission for Health Education Credentialing, Inc., is responsible for the CHES examination.

APPLICATION TO PATIENT/CONSUMER PROGRAMS

The COPA model directly addresses how educators in academic and practice settings need to change to prepare graduates for contemporary practice. In this section, the model is presented in the context of how patient/consumer programs need to change. Today, there are expectations that everyone is empowered to make health care decisions and be accountable. Patients and consumers need to prevent health problems, maintain the best levels of health possible, and be knowledgeable about treatments. Millions of Americans are living with and managing their chronic health problems. New health problems, such as childhood obesity, are emerging. Nurses and health professionals share responsibility for educating their patients and consumers. CBE is essential for patients and consumers. They need to actively participate in education programs and demonstrate they have the competencies needed to take care of themselves.

Setting: A large, urban clinic serves a diverse population. There are many different age groups, varied ethnic and cultural backgrounds, and a range of socioeconomic situations. The clinic staff reviews the clinic visit reports each month to determine patterns. They separate clients into same-diagnosis groups. Each month they look at different diagnoses. They are concerned because over 200 clients were seen in the clinic for problems related to controlling their diabetes. One hundred and fifty of the clients had completed the standard diabetes education course. All of them had between 8–10 clinic visits in the last three months, and 50 of the clients had completed the course twice.

Two staff members used CBE in previous work settings. They briefly shared the processes. Betty (RN) and John (PA) agree to gather more information and present it next month. They review the literature and find information about CBE, evidence-based practices, and current guidelines and standards. They organize the information according to the COPA model.

The American Diabetes Association Website (*http://www.diabetes. org/home.jsp*) has a large amount of information:

- Diabetes is a chronic disease that has no cure. There are an estimated 23.6 million children and adults in the United States, or 7.8% of the population, who have diabetes;
- An estimated 17.9 million have been diagnosed, about 5.7 million people are not aware they have the disease, and 57 million people have prediabetes;
- If the trend continues, one in three Americans and one in two minorities born in 2000 will develop diabetes in their lifetime;
- Each day, approximately 4,110 people are diagnosed with diabetes;
- In 2005, 1.5 million new cases of diabetes were diagnosed in people age 20 years and older;
- Heart disease and stroke account for about 65% of deaths in people with diabetes;
- Adults with diabetes have heart disease death rates about two to four times higher than adults without diabetes;
- The risk for stroke is 2 to 4 times higher, and the risk of death from stroke is 2.8 times higher, among people with diabetes;
- About 73% of adults with diabetes have blood pressure greater than or equal to 130/80 millimeters of mercury (mmHg) or use prescription medications for hypertension;
- Diabetic retinopathy causes 12,000 to 24,000 new cases of blindness each year, making diabetes the leading cause of new cases of blindness in adults 20–74 years of age;

- Diabetes is the leading cause of kidney failure, accounting for 44% of new cases in 2005;
- In 2005, 46,739 people with diabetes began treatment for end-stage renal disease (ESRD).

Question 1. What are the essential competencies and outcomes for managing health?

The American Diabetes Association (ADA) has developed the standards of care for persons with diabetes. The standards are based on numerous research studies. The recommendations are the best practices available for care. The standards address the major areas of management. The following are examples of ADA standards that the clinic must have in place:

- Medical care comes from a physician-coordinated team and may include, but is not limited to, physicians, nurse practitioners, physician's assistants, nurses, dietitians, pharmacists, and mental health professionals with expertise and a special interest in diabetes;
- Management plan is individualized and there are therapeutic partnerships among the patient and family, the physician, and other members of the health care team;
- It is essential in this collaborative and integrated team approach that individuals with diabetes assume an active role in their care;
- A variety of strategies and techniques are needed to provide adequate education and development of problem-solving skills in the various aspects of diabetes management;
- Management plan requires that each aspect is understood and agreed on by the patient and the care providers;
- Diabetes self-management education (DSME) as an integral component of care. In developing the plan, consideration should be given to the patient's age, school or work schedule and conditions, physical activity, eating patterns, social situation and personality, cultural factors, and presence of complications of diabetes or other medical conditions.

The clinic has the major responsibility of creating an environment that is supportive and has the knowledge and resources to share with its clients.

Table 3.5

CONGRUENCE OF LENBURG'S CORE COMPETENCIES AND ADA STANDARDS

CORE COMPETENCIES	ADA STANDARDS
Assessment and Intervention Skills	For a variety of reasons, some people with diabetes and their health care providers do not achieve the desired goals of treatment. Rethinking the treatment regimen may require assessment of barriers to adherence including income, educational attainment, and competing demands, including those related to family responsibilities and family dynamics.
Communication Skills	Record all values. Accurately interpret what the values mean. Use the data to adjust food intake, exercise, or pharmacological therapy to achieve specific glycemic goals.
Critical Thinking Skills	A variety of strategies and techniques are needed to provide adequate education and develop problem-solving skills in the various aspects of diabetes management.
Human Caring and Relationship Skills	Using the patient–provider relationship as a foundation for further treatment can increase the likelihood that the patient will accept referral for other services. It is important to establish that emotional well-being is part of diabetes management.
Management Skills	Individual client management plan.
Leadership Skills	Clients take an active role and collaborate with team members.
Teaching Skills	Diabetes self-management education (DSME) as an integral component of care.

Lenburg's (1999) eight core competencies are extended to include persons with diabetes. Generally, the focus of the model is on the programs developed by educators. In this scenario, the learners, persons with diabetes, need to educate themselves and manage their disease. Table 3.5 demonstrates the congruence between Lenburg's Core Competencies and ADA Standards.

A sample list of competencies is developed, based on ADA practice standards. The competencies are examples of some of the areas targeted. At the end of the DSME program, the clients will be able to:

- Determine specific actions related to results of psychosocial screening (attitudes about the illness; expectations for medical management and outcomes; affect/mood; general and diabetes-related quality of life; resources; financial, social, and emotional status, and psychiatric history);
- Correctly demonstrate self-monitoring of blood glucose (SMBG) at least three times a day if they use multiple insulin injections or insulin pump therapy;
- Record all values;
- Accurately interpret what the values mean;
- Use the data to adjust food intake, exercise, or pharmacological therapy to achieve specific glycemic goals;
- Integrate principles of Medical Nutrition Therapy (MNT) into their self-management plan;
- Choose physical activities and behavior-modification strategies to lose and maintain weight;
- Practice self-management behavior changes recommended in DSME;
- Participate in the continuing measurement and monitoring as specified in DSME.

Question 2. What are indicators that define the competencies?

The indicators for each of the competencies should be specific and only include the actions and responses essential for carrying it out (Lenburg, 1999). Table 3.6 matches a sample of the competencies to critical elements (indicators).

Once the competencies and critical elements (indicators) are determined, specific learning activities are selected. Step 3 in the COPA model addresses how to determine the most effective ways to learn competencies.

Question 3. What are the most effective ways to learn the competencies?

In this scenario, the clients are developing self-management skills for their diabetes. The clients are educating themselves. The materials and information provided and available to the clients need to be understand-

Table 3.6

SAMPLE COMPETENCIES AND CRITICAL ELEMENTS (INDICATORS)

SAMPLE COMPETENCIES	CRITICAL ELEMENTS (INDICATORS)
Determine specific actions related to results of psychosocial screening (attitudes about the illness; expectations for medical management and outcomes; affect/mood; general and diabetes-related quality of life; resources; financial, social, emotional status, and psychiatric history).	Participate in group or individual sessions focused on attitudes about diabetes. Complete psychosocial screening at the end of the sessions. Evaluate whether changes in attitudes are more positive than previous screening. If needed, participate in smoking cessation counseling. Select and follow a smoking cessation treatment plan. Choose the services of a community health worker to provide additional support.
Correctly demonstrate self-monitoring of blood glucose (SMBG) at least three times a day if they use multiple insulin injections or insulin pump therapy.	Use clean technique to cleanse site. Select an appropriate site to get blood sample. Correctly follow the directions of the meter. Accurately read the results. Record date, time, and results of the test.
Integrate principles of Medical Nutrition Therapy (MNT) into their self-management plan.	Arrange sessions with a registered dietitian (RD) to determine appropriate elements of MNT for you. Collaborate with the RD to develop nutrition interventions based on your age, type of diabetes, pharmacological treatment, lipid levels, and other medical conditions. Monitor dietary intake, weight, physical activities, glucose levels, blood pressure, and lipid levels as recommended. Collaborate with RD to modify MNT to find new ways to reach unmet goals and maintain goals being met.
Choose physical activities and behavior-modification strategies to lose and maintain weight.	Select one or more physical activities that are congruent with your abilities and behaviors. Participate in moderate-intensity physical activities at least 30 minutes on most, ideally all, days of the week. Measure level of activity so it is at 50%–70% of maximum heart rate. When not contraindicated, persons with type 2 diabetes should perform resistance training three times per week.

Adapted from Lenburg (1999).

able and useful. The clinic staff has the responsibility to help clients educate themselves.

The Institute of Medicine (2004) identified that half of adults in America lack the literacy and numerical skills to find, integrate, and apply patient education materials. It is essential that clients gain knowledge from the material and actually change health behaviors.

Clients are expected to assume greater responsibility for their own health care. They need to actively participate in their care, especially for those with chronic diseases such as diabetes and obesity. It is critical to focus on a few key concepts when helping persons with low literacy to understand educational materials. Another strategy to promote self-education is to have clients evaluate the education materials and make suggestions for improvements (Siegel, Rhinehart, Jackson, & Chiarello, 2006). Paying attention to literacy levels will make a positive difference in the ability of clients to manage their own care.

The most effective way for clients to learn the competencies is to provide multiple options. Suggestions are to provide learning resources and activities with:

- Appropriate literacy levels;
- Attention to cultural habits, values, and beliefs;
- Options for low- to high-technology methods;
- Individual and collaborative group self-directed learning opportunities;
- Observation and demonstration of various types of skills;
- A steady, manageable pace of information sharing;
- Learning materials to keep for additional review and practice;
- Timely and comprehensive feedback on performance;
- Ongoing support and guidance to clarify and verify knowledge, skills, and beliefs (Mitchell, 2004).

Some competencies, such as checking blood glucose, injecting insulin, and managing an insulin pump, require practice and demonstration. The client can also explain the "why" of what they are doing. Additionally, a scenario which requires the client to make decisions about care in given situations is useful.

Achieving behavioral competencies can be done through reflection and group discussion. Clients can support each other and offer solutions related to living with diabetes, maintaining glucose levels, menus, and exercise.

Physical activity competencies are demonstrated by the selected activities and documentation of what was done each day. Reflection and journaling on which activities were most helpful and doable, which ones caused health problems, and which ones helped achieve the best results can be useful.

One strategy to help clients become competent is for clinic staff to help them develop an action plan. An action plan contains short-term goals to start the process of immediate behavior changes. An example related to physical activity is a client's decision to walk six blocks each day before watching television in the evening. An action plan starts the process of doing things to achieve goals. As goals are met, the plan is revised and extended to include new activities. A vital aspect of an action plan is that clients are in control of making decisions, they select options for achieving and demonstrating competence, and become empowered to care for themselves (Siegel, Rhinehart, Jackson, & Chiarello, 2006). The last step in the model is creating examinations and assessments.

Question 4. What are the most effective ways to document that learners have achieved the required competencies?

The ADA has very specific standards not only for care, but for individual outcomes. Persons with diabetes can demonstrate competence in managing their disease through a variety of measures:

- Maintain a daily normal (nondiabetic) blood glucose level, between 70 and 130 mg/dl before meals, and less than 180 two hours after starting a meal;
- Maintain an A1C (glycated hemoglobin or HbA1c) value of 7% or less;
- Achieve and maintain a normal body weight;
- Perform and document at least 150 minutes/week of moderate-intensity aerobic physical activity (50–70% of maximum heart rate);
- Psychosocial screening and follow-up behaviors are within normal ranges;

- A systolic blood pressure of <130 mmHg and a diastolic blood pressure of <80 mmHg are within normal limits;
- Lipid values (LDL cholesterol <100 mg/dl, HDL cholesterol >50 mg/dl, and triglycerides <150 mg/dl) are within normal limits;
- Documentation of aspirin therapy (75–162 mg/day);
- Quit smoking or in a cessation program;
- Normal results from comprehensive foot screenings;
- Normal results from comprehensive eye examinations.

The information above is then matched with the selected competencies. When the values are within normal limits, the client is competent to provide self-care and maintain the best health possible.

Example of an Application in a Client/Consumer Education Program

The Agency for Healthcare Research and Quality (AHRQ) has developed *Diabetes Care Quality Improvement: A Resource Guide for State Action* and its companion workbook, *Diabetes Care Quality Improvement: A Workbook for State Action*. These materials were designed in partnership with the Council of State Governments to help states assess the quality of diabetes care and create quality-improvement strategies. States can make changes in health care delivery and best practices that can transform health care systems, reduce costs, and improve public health. For specific diseases like diabetes, a number of states already have substantial programs underway that can shape and inform the development of new initiatives. To assist such efforts, AHRQ has released the following products, developed in consultation with diabetes control and prevention experts at all levels:

- *Diabetes Care Quality Improvement: A Resource Guide for State Action*. This comprehensive guide offers a wealth of information and details for a range of participants in a state's quality-improvement effort, including state-elected leaders, executive branch officials, and other nongovernmental state and local health care leaders. The *Resource Guide* provides background information, analysis of state and national data, and guidance for developing a state quality-improvement plan. It gives an extensive listing of many ongoing national, state, and local efforts to improve diabetes care quality.'

■ *Diabetes Care Quality Improvement: A Workbook for State Action.* A companion to the *Resource Guide*, the interactive *Workbook* presents review exercises for state leaders on the key skills and lessons from the *Resource Guide* to use in implementing health care quality improvement plans in their states. These practical exercises enable *Workbook* users to focus on their states in comparison to the nation and other states. The resources are available for download at: http://www.ahrq.gov/QUAL/diabqualoc.htm.

SUMMARY

The COPA is a framework for determining the elements of a program or course. The model is comprehensive, and includes:

■ Deciding essential competencies for practice;
■ The indicators of competencies;
■ Effective ways to learn competencies;
■ Efficient ways to document that the learners have achieved them.

Competencies are arranged under Lenburg's eight core practice competencies. Traditional behavioral objectives are transformed into outcome statements. The purpose of outcome statements is to determine whether learners have attained the competencies necessary to begin practicing in their discipline. The scenarios focus on three different types of educational programs: academic, staff development, and client/consumer. Examples of how CBE has been applied to the educational programs in the scenarios are included. Chapter 4 focuses on the actual development of competency statements, how to write them, and decisions about how to measure them.

CHAPTER 3 ACTIVITY

Chapters 1 and 2 provided a foundation for developing a CBE program or course. Depending on your setting and goals, you have the essential information to begin development. This chapter provides general information and examples of how to use the COPA model. Review your activities from the two previous chapters. Answer the four questions

Exhibit 3.1

ESSENTIAL QUESTIONS	RESPONSES TO QUESTIONS
■ What are the essential competencies and outcomes for contemporary practice? ■ What are the indicators that define those competencies? ■ What are the most effective ways to learn those competencies? ■ What are the most effective ways to document that learners and/or practitioners have achieved the required competencies?	

Adapted from Lenburg (1999).

posed in Exhibit 3.1 to further develop your CBE program or course. You do not have to include the competency statements until you complete chapter 4.

REFERENCES

Adkins, S. (2004). Beneath the tip of the iceberg. *Training + Development, 58*(2), 28–33. Retrieved December 10, 2008, from MasterFILE Premier database.

Bastable, S. B. (2003). *Nurses as educators: Principles of teaching and learning for nursing practice.* Sudbury, MA: Jones and Bartlett.

Clark, C. C. (2009). *Creative nursing leadership & management.* Sudbury, MA: Jones and Bartlett.

Dettmer, P. (2006). New blooms in established fields: Four domains of learning and doing. *Roeper Review, 28*(2), 70–78. Retrieved December 10, 2008, from MasterFILE Premier database.

Institute of Medicine. (2004). *Health Literacy: A prescription to end confusion.* Washington, DC: National Academies.

Lenburg, C. B. (1999). The framework, concepts, and methods of the competency outcomes and performance assessment (COPA) model. *Online Journal of Issues in Nursing, 4*(3). Retrieved December 15, 2008, from http://www.nursingworld.org/ojin

Mager, R. (1975). *Preparing instructional objectives.* Belmont, CA: Fearon.

McKeachie, W. J., & Svinicki, M. (2006). *Teaching tips: Strategies, research, and theories for college and university teachers*. Boston: Houghton Mifflin.

Mitchell, G. (2004). Adult learning and high-stakes testing: Strategies for success. *Adult Learning, 15*(3/4), 16–18.

National Commisssion for Health Education Credentialing, Inc. (NCHEC). Retrieved October 29, 2008, from http//nchec.cyzap.net/aboutnhec/mission/

Siegel, J. D., Rhinehart, E., Jackson, M., & Chiarello, L. (2006). Management of multi-drug-resistant organisms in healthcare settings. Atlanta, GA: Centers for Disease Control and Prevention. Retrieved February 1, 2009, from http://www.cdc.gov/ncidod/dhqp/pdf/ar/MDROGuideline2006.pdf

Seligman, H. K., Wallace, A. S., DeWalt, D. A., Sehillinger, D., Arnold, C. L., Shilliday, B. B., et al. (2007). Facilitating behavior change with low-literacy patient education materials. *American Journal of Health Behavior, 7*(31) (Suppl.1), S69–S78.

Soule, B. (2009). *Top issues in infection prevention and control for 2009*. Oakbrook, IL: Joint Commission on Accreditation of Healthcare Organizations. Retrieved February 1, 2009, from http://www.jcrinc.com/Top-Issues-in-Infection-Prevention-and-Control-for-2009/

Steltzer, T. M. (Ed.). (2003). *Five keys to successful nursing management*. Philadelphia: Lippincott Williams Wilkins.

Weimer, M. (2002). *Learner-centered teaching*. San Francisco: Jossey Bass.

Wright, D. (2005). *The ultimate guide to competency assessment in healthcare*. Minneapolis, MN: Creative Health Care Management, Inc.

ADDITIONAL RESOURCES

The following sites provide examples of CBE programs or courses.

Boston Healing Landscape Project is a site for cultural competency in U.S. health care with best practice Website recommendations, *http://www.bu.edu/bhlp/pages/resources/cultural_competency/ education.html*

The National Center for Education Statistics (NCES) is the primary federal entity for collecting, analyzing, and reporting data related to education in the United States and other nations. It fulfills a congressional mandate to collect, collate, analyze, and report full and complete statistics on the condition of education in the United States; conduct and publish reports and specialized analyses of the meaning and significance of such statistics; assist state and local education agencies in improving their statistics systems; and review and report on education activities in foreign countries: http://nces.ed.gov/pubs2002/2002159.pdf

Defining and Assessing Learning: Exploring Competency-Based Initiatives. Prepared for the Council of the National Postsecondary Education Cooperative (NPEC) and its Working Group on Competency-Based Initiatives by Elizabeth A. Jones and Richard A. Voorhees, with Karen Paulson. (2002). Washington, DC: U.S. Department of Education. Available at http://nces.ed.gov/pubsearch/pubsinfo.asp? pubid-2002175

National Commission for Health Education Credentialing, Inc. (NCHEC)
http://nchec.cyzap.net/aboutnchec/mission/

NCHEC's mission is to improve the practice of health education and to serve the public and profession of health education by certifying health-education specialists, promoting professional development, and strengthening professional preparation and practice. The major purposes of NCHEC are:

■ Development and administration of a national competency-based examination;
■ Development of standards for professional preparation;
■ Professional development through continuing education programs.

National Eye Health Education Program Five-Year Agenda
http://www.nei.nih.gov/nehep/research/
Effective_Education_to_Target_Populations.pdf

Effective Education to Target Populations research was conducted to gain a better understanding of the most effective ways to deliver eye health messages to target populations, and the most appropriate settings for these messages to reach their audiences. In addition to the in-house research, a literature review was conducted to learn more about the cultural and communication issues that face these populations, and the most current accepted and proven practices that have worked in the delivery of health education and promotion messages.

The Indian Health Service (IHS) Integrated Best Practice Model. Basic Diabetes Care and Education: A Systems Approach
http://www.betterdiabetescare.nih.gov/NEEDSbestpracticemodel.htm

This site contains information about determining needs and setting priorities for systems change and provides a tool for a best practice model.

Transitioning to the CBE Approach

JANICE L. McCOY

OVERVIEW

This chapter addresses the development of competency statements for three different groups: learners in educational programs, staff, and patients/consumers. The use of current standards of practice, regulatory requirements, and employer and consumer expectations is explored. How to change current objectives to competency statements is discussed, including creating learning statements/activities that lead to completion of competencies. Decisions about the type of assessments (objective or performance) to use in measuring competencies/learning statements are examined.

INTRODUCTION

Competency can be described as possessing the skills, understanding, and supporting values needed to function safely and independently. Definitions of competent performance will vary with populations. For example, competent performance for health care providers will be different from that for patients/consumers. Competency statements must accurately express the outcome expectations for a specified population.

Determining what constitutes competent performance is critical for achieving outstanding outcomes. Developing competency statements that are unrealistic will result in competent learners being deemed incompetent. The opposite is true if competency statements are established at too low a level: incompetent learners will be deemed competent. Identifying the midpoint on the novice-expert continuum for a given population may be a starting point. Adjustments up or down can be made based on learner population and level of competency desired.

HOW TO WRITE COMPETENCY STATEMENTS

Well-written competency statements are the key to identifying the knowledge, skills, and attitudes desired. According to Lenburg (1999), the greatest hurdle that must be overcome is continuing to embrace the traditional view of using behavioral objectives as the only acceptable format for learning and practice. Having a clear understanding of the difference between objectives and competencies is crucial in order to make the transition from objectives to competencies. Competency outcomes look at the end results: the knowledge, skills, and behaviors expected for practice or to manage personal well-being. Behavioral objectives as currently used focus on learning content, and may not reflect practice or health maintenance expectations.

Competency statements must be in line with current practice standards and employer/consumer expectations. For consumers, competency statements must also reflect their need to manage personal health and well-being. For this to happen, input from multiple stakeholders must occur. Appropriate and accurate competencies cannot be created if one group is unaware of the expectations of other major stakeholders. Regulatory agencies, employers, faculty, and consumers must have a say in what constitutes competent performance. To begin the process of changing to competency statements, it is necessary to identify and assemble stakeholders from education, practice, regulation, and consumers.

Chapter 3 presented Lenburg's (1999) Competency Outcomes and Performance Assessment (COPA) model and introduced four questions to guide conversion to competency outcome statements. Using Lenburg's four questions and any subcomponents of the questions requires a step-by-step process, and will help stakeholders change perspective from traditional behavioral objectives to competency outcome statements. Two major components are also identified to assist in answering the first question.

Slight modifications of the first of Lenburg's four questions make them applicable to continuing competence and consumer education.

Question 1

- **Education:** "What are the essential competencies and outcomes for contemporary practice that a new graduate must possess?" (Lenburg, 1999, p. 3).

    1. What are the required competencies?
    2. Are they worded as practice-based outcomes and not as traditional behavioral objectives?
- **Continuing competence:** What are the essential competencies and outcomes for continuing practice?

    1. What are the required competencies of the setting?
    2. Are they worded as practice-based outcomes and not as traditional behavioral objectives?
- **Consumer education:** What are the essential competencies and outcomes for consumer self-management of health?

    1. What are the required competencies for the specific consumer health issue?
    2. Are they worded as practice-based outcomes and not as traditional behavioral objectives?

Stakeholders must first identify the desired competencies for contemporary practice (initial entry or continuing) or consumer education. Once the desired competencies are known, alignment is made between the desired competencies, the major content areas of any existing curricula, education standards, Lenburg's (1999) eight core competencies, practice expectations, regulations, or patient teaching materials (where applicable).

Education

Program faculty typically answer Question 1 based on The Essentials for Baccalaureate Education for Professional Nursing Practice (American

Association of Colleges in Nursing [AACN], 1998) that lists the desired knowledge and skills to be acquired. Unfortunately, the skills and knowledge, as presented, are written in traditional behavioral objective format and when incorporated into a curriculum, the behavioral objective format is usually repeated. Together, faculty and stakeholders must align the major areas from The Essentials for Baccalaureate Education for Professional Nursing Practice (AACN, 1998) with the list of desired competencies for contemporary practice.

Next, faculty and stakeholders should compare Lenburg's (1999) core competencies with the list of desired competencies for contemporary practice and the placement of knowledge and skills from The Essentials for Baccalaureate Education for Professional Nursing Practice. The goal is to align the desired competencies with required program standards, regulatory requirements, and practice expectations. Once this alignment has occurred, additional review by the group may identify overlooked competencies or subskills. Additional competency categories and/or subskills under existing categories can be added at this time.

The final step in answering the first question is to review the wording of each competency statement. Competency statements focus on outcomes: the knowledge and skills the learner must use in practice. Competency statements should focus on the learner and the essential competence (cognitive, affective, or psychomotor) to be realized at the conclusion of the learning period.

Continuing Competency

The competency of health care staff is essential to the delivery of high-quality patient care (Alspach, 2008). Whelan (2006) advises that one of the greatest challenges within a changing health care environment is ensuring a competent nursing staff to care for patients. When identifying competencies, staff developers must recognize the dynamic nature of contemporary practice. Practice expectations change as new information, technologies, or practice challenges surface. Staff developers must examine current practice competency requirements, but also look to what competencies may be required in the future. Once again, input from stakeholders is essential to identifying the essential competencies.

Outside agencies, such as The Joint Commission (formerly know as The Joint Commission on the Accreditation of Healthcare Organizations

[JCAHO]), look at staff competence and define competency (The Joint Commission, 2005). The Joint Commission requires that clinical competence be assessed, and holds institutional leaders accountable for ensuring that competency is assessed, maintained, demonstrated, and continually improved (Redman, Lenburg, & Hinton-Walker, 2008). In addition, competency expectations change as nursing staff is realigned to different areas, so continuing competence must address staff along the novice-to-expert continuum.

Comparing national patient safety goals with internal data may uncover the need for certain competencies. During the process, competencies may surface that are nice to possess but not essential to the job. The challenge is to narrow the list of essential competencies down to no more than 10 for any given time period. Wright (2005) stresses that the selected competencies should only include those that are needed by every employee in a specified practice area. A sample online worksheet, developed by Wright (2005), will assist in identifying continuing competency. Stakeholders should also review Lenburg's (1999) core competencies, because more experienced staff may have higher expectations and desire higher level core competencies. The goal is to align the desired competencies with required standards.

Consumer Education

Patient educators are guided by health care expectations of consumers. As consumers assume a more proactive role in their health, demand for understandable and accurate information increases. A consequence of people living longer is the increasing prevalence of chronic diseases. In addition, with the movement of care to the community and the push for self-responsibility for health and well-being, consumers are demanding information in order to maintain health or manage a given disease (acute and chronic). Consumers want to be involved in decisions about their health, but need information in order to make informed decisions.

As stated previously, stakeholders need to be identified. Possible stakeholders are from consumer education, practice, patient advocacy organizations, health information organizations, and consumer groups. Identifying competencies is more involved because consumer education must address specific areas such as acute or chronic illnesses, wellness activities, health maintenance/management, specific skills (e.g., injections, dressing changes, wound management), etc. Because of the almost endless list of major content areas, identifying only the essential competencies for a specific area is crucial. Patient education materials already exist for many of the areas, and can be used to align desired competencies.

Whether the competency statement is for education, continuing competence, or consumer education, following some general rules will assist in the conversion from traditional behavioral objectives to competency-oriented outcomes. Each competency statement should:

- Begin with a stem that is oriented to the learner's action.
  - ○ **Education**: All stems in *The Essentials for Baccalaureate Education for Professional Nursing Practice* (AACN, 1998) read, "Course work or clinical experiences should provide the graduate with the knowledge and skills to...." The focus is on course work and clinical experiences providing knowledge and skills, not on what the learner should demonstrate. A more correct stem would be, "At the conclusion of the course (module, unit, etc.), the learner will be able to..." The focus with this stem is on the learner's ability to demonstrate a practice-related essential at the conclusion of the learning unit.
  - ○ **Continuing competence**: The position description within many organizations is viewed as the expectations the employer has for the employee at the time of hire. Position descriptions vary greatly in detail and may not clearly state the core competencies required for the position, yet these descriptions are used to evaluate employees annually. Although organizations must be dynamic and responsive to changing environments, using initial employment position descriptions to measure competence does not allow for changes within the organization or practice and staff development. Continuing competence requires a review of expectations as the external and internal environments change, adjusting expectations accordingly. Expectations must clearly state the essential performance the staff person must demonstrate 100% of the time.
  - ○ **Consumer education**: As with any educational offering, the competency statement for consumers must focus on the

learner and not on the content. Although there may be necessary content a consumer needs to know for a specific health care issue, the focus must be on what is essential for the consumer to be able to do with the information. Adult learners need to see the relevance in learning something new and be able to apply new knowledge immediately. Understanding the importance of changing behavior encourages the individual to choose change. Unlike learners in higher education and continuing competence, consumers can choose to not become competent in personal health care concerns without the fear of scholastic or employment consequences.

■ Precisely state what results are to be attained for each competency: what the learner should be able to do at the conclusion of the learning unit.
  ○ **Education**: *The Essentials for Baccalaureate Education for Professional Nursing Practice* identifies what each content area should include, but does not precisely state the essential competency the learner must demonstrate at the conclusion of the learning unit. The Essentials Statements name the knowledge and understanding the learner must possess for each content area.
  ○ **Continuing competence**: Continuing education offerings are often used to demonstrate continuing competency. The problem is that the typical continuing education offering focuses on *knowing* or *knowing how to do* something, not on actually performing the action. Continuing education offerings can be used if a follow-up assessment activity measures application to real-world practice situations.
  ○ **Consumer education**: Most patient teaching situations involve teaching a skill or changing a behavior. Competencies involving skills should require the consumer to perform the skill. The focus of return demonstration is consistent with *doing* rather than *knowing how to do* a skill. Behavioral change competencies are dependent on the consumer choosing to change a behavior. Although the competencies may clearly state what behavior is expected, the consumer may choose not to change and never achieve the expected outcome. The consumer would stop at the *know* or *know how to do* stage by choice.

■ Include the essential competency to be achieved by the end of the learning period. What is the expected level of competence at the end of the course (module, unit, etc.)? The expectations for a beginning learner may differ from those of advanced learners.

○ **Education**: The exit competencies for an educational program will express the expected outcomes at program completion. The individual program course competencies may begin with lower-level expectations that increase in complexity until the program competencies are achieved. Competencies reflect the learning level, which spans small units to whole programs.

○ **Continuing competence**: Smaller learning units typically occur within organizations. Installation of a new phone system may require new skills. The essential skills needed to operate the new phone system must be identified and communicated clearly for all employees.

○ **Consumer education**: Competency identification for consumer education can be challenging, as the population is very diverse. Health maintenance or improvement competencies must consider, age, current physical and mental health status, educational level, language, cultural beliefs, etc. A one-size-fits-all approach may not be the most effective way to assure competence in personal health issues. Essential competencies can be identified, but they may need to be individualized in order to achieve desired outcomes.

■ Present each competency statement clearly and concisely so readers easily understand the action expected.

○ **Education**: *The Essentials for Baccalaureate Education for Professional Nursing Practice* contains a statement defining assessment, but does not clearly and concisely state the expected outcomes for assessment activities. The statement can be modified to read, *Provide care to individuals, families, communities, or populations based on collecting, analyzing, and synthesizing health data, data-driven nursing judgments, and evaluation of care outcomes.* The modified statement clearly indicates the expected behavior the learner must demonstrate.

○ **Continuing competence**: Because position descriptions are used to communicate job expectations upon entry, they need to be stated in a manner that is understandable to all readers.

The statements should not be open to interpretation by the reader. The creators of the position description have certain performance expectations, and must clearly communicate their expectations in the position description.

○ **Consumer education**: Consumers also need to understand the actions expected. Competency statements that are not clear and concise can lead to confusion about how and what should be performed.

■ Begin each statement with a verb that describes the expected outcome at the appropriate level for the learner population. Behavioral objectives use verbs from one of the taxonomies. Verbs for higher level learning assume that lower level learning has occurred in order to achieve the higher level function. Competency outcomes are action oriented, therefore, action verbs must be used. The verbs must reflect what is expected in practice. Understanding or knowing how to do something is not enough. The learner must be able to actually perform the action according to practice expectations. Action verbs should be selected at or above the application level.

○ **Education**: Verbs for the application level may be more prevalent at the beginning of an educational program, but as learners progress through the courses, verbs designed to demonstrate analysis and synthesis will increase. Using real-world practice situations assists learners in seeing the relevance to actual practice.

○ **Continuing competence**: Verbs for higher levels are usually used for demonstrating continuing competence. Experienced staff should be able to demonstrate analysis and synthesis in real-world practice situations.

○ **Consumer education**: Verbs for application should be the lowest level used.

■ Write the competency statement so it is consistent with current standards and contemporary practice expectations.

○ **Education**: Content experts from practice and regulation are invaluable for critiquing competency statements for congruency between the statement and current standards and contemporary practice expectations. Using experts from practice and regulation contributes to narrowing the gap between education and practice, thus assisting faculty to prepare graduates for the workplace.

○ **Continuing competence**: External and internal factors influence workplace and practice environments. Regulatory agencies revise their expectations periodically and new standards of practice may surface. Different practice areas may have different standards of practice. Organizations may change philosophy and purpose. Competency statements must reflect the internal and external forces pushing the change.

○ **Consumer education**: Health care information and technology is changing rapidly; therefore, consumer information must be carefully selected for use in any consumer education program. Competency statements for consumer education must be consistent with current standards. Statements must also reflect a level of performance that is safe and realistic for the consumer.

■ Limit competency statements to those that contribute to achieving the expected overall performance outcomes. It is critical at this point to discriminate between what would be nice vs. what is absolutely necessary to meet the expectations of multiple stakeholders. The available time for learning may be limited; therefore, competencies must be achievable within the time allowed.

○ **Education**: *The Essentials of Baccalaureate Education for Professional Nursing Practice* delineates the essential content for baccalaureate nursing programs. Practice and regulatory experts can identify competencies that are essential for current practice. The two must be blended to reflect only the essential competencies required for contemporary practice.

○ **Continuing competence**: In any workplace, there are numerous areas where improvement in performance could be beneficial. The key is to focus on the competencies needed within the organization and practice at a given point in time. Wright (2005) has developed a worksheet to help identify the essential competencies needed. Using this worksheet will help focus on the competencies that will have the greatest effect on outcomes. Wright (2005) suggests limiting competencies to 10 or less, and they should be confined to those skills required by 100% of the employees in the job class.

○ **Consumer education**: As with all competency statements, identifying the essential competencies is the key to implementing a successful competence-based education program. Consumer education program developers must be careful to include only essential competencies, otherwise the learner may be overwhelmed. Competency statements should focus on overall performance by consumers to maintain or improve health status.

Examples using the previous steps for performance-based competency statements for education, continuing competence, and consumer education are:

■ **Education Example**: At the conclusion of the learning unit, the learner will be able to use outcome measures to evaluate effectiveness of care;
■ **Continuing Competency Example**: At the conclusion of the learning unit, the learner will be able to use evaluative statements when charting to communicate progress toward meeting identified patient outcomes;
■ **Consumer Education Example**: At the conclusion of the learning unit, the learner will be able to self-administer insulin using correct injection technique, site selection, and dose.

Each statement:

■ Focuses on the learner;
■ Precisely states what results are expected;
■ Includes an essential competency to achieve;
■ Has a common meaning;
■ Is leveled according to the learner population;
■ Is consistent with current standards;
■ Is a necessary competency for achieving overall performance outcomes.

WRITING LEARNING STATEMENTS THAT LEAD TO COMPETENT PERFORMANCE

Competency statements identify the expected outcomes at the conclusion of a learning period (see Table 4.1). The next step in converting to a competency-based process is to answer Lenburg's (1999, p. 3)

Table 4.1

CHANGING TO A COMPETENCY FRAMEWORK

Identifying desired competencies	Project leader selects a group of stakeholders from education, practice, regulation, and consumers.
	Stakeholders create a list of desired competencies for contemporary practice or consumer education.
	Stakeholders align current major content areas with the list of desired competencies for contemporary practice or consumer education. Major content areas could come from curricula, continuing education modules, or patient education materials.
	Stakeholders align Lenburg's (1999) core competencies (or core competencies for consumer education) with the list of desired competencies for contemporary practice (or consumer education needs).
	Stakeholders align the major areas:
	■ Education: *The Essentials for Baccalaureate Education for Professional Nursing Practice* (AACN, 1998) with the list of desired competencies for contemporary practice and regulatory agency requirements;
	■ Continuing Competence: Best practices, practice standards, certification competencies, and regulatory agency regulations;
	■ Consumer Education: Existing consumer teaching materials.
	Stakeholders review the list of desired competencies, adding/deleting as indicated.
Developing competency statements for each desired competency	Each competency statement must focus on what the learner must demonstrate. Begin each competency statement with: "At the conclusion of the course (module, unit, etc.), the learner will be able to":
	Precisely state what results are to be attained for each competency; what should the learner be able to do. The focus is to move from *knowing* and *knowing how* to actually *doing*.
	Include the essential competency to be achieved by the end of the learning period. What is the expected level of competence at the end of the course (module, unit, etc.)?
	State each competency statement clearly and concisely so multiple readers easily understand the action expected.
	Begin each statement with a verb that describes the expected outcome at the appropriate level for the learner population.
	Write the competency statement so it is consistent with current standards and expectations for education, continuing competence, or consumer education.
	Limit competency statements to those that contribute to achieving the expected overall performance outcomes. Discriminate between what would be nice vs. what is necessary.

second question, "What are the indicators that define those competencies?" The indicators, when taken as a whole, articulate the expected competence in specific terms.

To guide learners, each competency must be broken down into the essential behaviors required to meet the competency. These essential behaviors are referred to as *indicators*, and are the critical elements required for demonstrating competency in a given skill or behavior. Critical elements are a "set of single, discrete, observable behaviors" (Lenburg, 1999). Critical elements represent those principles essential to competent performance; they are not steps in a procedure.

The following general guidelines will assist in identifying and developing the indicators (essential behaviors) for each competency statement:

- Specific indicators need to be identified that clearly define each competency. The indicators should include only the essential behaviors required to be deemed competent for actual practice. When all indicators for a given competency are taken collectively, they clearly define the expected competence. Using the competency statements given previously, examples of possible indicators are:
  - ○ **Education Example of Indicators**: At the conclusion of the learning unit, the learner will be able to use outcome measures to evaluate effectiveness of care:
    1. Data collection;
    2. Data analysis;
    3. Using effectiveness criteria;
    4. Comparing expected outcomes with actual outcomes;
    5. Judging effectiveness based on data;
    6. Recommendation.

  - ○ **Continuing Competency Example of Indicators**: At the conclusion of the learning unit, the learner will be able to use evaluative statements when charting to communicate progress toward meeting identified patient outcomes:
    1. Data analysis;
    2. Writing evaluative statements based on data;
    3. Comparing expected outcomes with actual outcomes;
    4. Judging effectiveness based on data.

○ **Consumer Education Example of Indicators**: At the conclusion of the learning unit, the learner will be able to self-administer insulin using correct injection technique, site selection, and dose:

1. Identifying prescribed medication;
2. Site preparation/rotation;
3. Injection procedure;
4. Documentation.

The above indicators are only a list of essential behaviors, and they need to be further developed into meaningful learning statements. The next step is to add verbs from one of the learning taxonomies (cognitive, affective, and psychomotor). This will move the critical element closer to being an actual indicator.

Each critical element should begin with a verb similar to traditional behavioral objectives. The acceptable verbs are listed in one of the taxonomies for the affective, psychomotor, or cognitive domains. The Adams Center for Teaching Excellence (2005) explains the affective, psychomotor, or cognitive taxonomies, and provides examples for each level of the three common taxonomies.

Using the previous competency statements and the first critical element, acceptable verbs for indicators are:

■ **Education Example**: At the conclusion of the learning unit, the learner will be able to use outcome measures to evaluate effectiveness of care:

1. Data collection (first critical element)

   ● Create a data collection plan to include:
     ❑ A brief description of the project;
     ❑ Specific data that are needed;
     ❑ Rationale for collecting the data;
     ❑ What insight the data might provide;
     ❑ How it will help effectiveness of care;
     ❑ What will be done with the data once it has been collected?
   ● Design data-collection methodologies to include:

❑ How many observations are needed?

❑ What time interval should be part of the study;

❑ Whether past, present, and future data will be collected;

❑ Methodologies that will be employed to record all the data.

■ **Continuing Competency Example**: At the conclusion of the learning unit, the learner will be able to use evaluative statements when charting to communicate progress toward meeting identified patient outcomes:

1. Data analysis (first critical element)

● Interpret patient care data by:
   ❑ Accessing patient data using facility health care information system;
   ❑ Selecting, sorting, and summarizing patient care data;
   ❑ Transforming patient care data into information;
   ❑ Transforming patient care information into knowledge.

■ **Consumer Education Example**: At the conclusion of the learning unit, the learner will be able to self-administer insulin using correct injection technique, site selection, and dose:

1. Medication identification (first critical element)

● Examine insulin prescription:
   ❑ Identify type prescribed;
   ❑ Identify time to be administered;
   ❑ Identify number of units prescribed.
● Compare insulin prescription to insulin vial:
   ❑ Verify type prescribed;
   ❑ State process if discrepancies exist.
● Assess usability of insulin:
   ❑ Assess appearance based on type;
   ❑ Select mixing procedure based on type;
   ❑ State conditions for when to discard.

■ The learning statement verb must identify the performance at the high end of the performance level desired:

1. **Education Example**: The verbs used in the previous Education example are at the synthesis level in the cognitive domain.

Synthesis is a high-end performance level and an expectation for Baccalaureate Education;

2. **Continuing Competency Example**: The verbs used in the previous Continuing Competency example range from the analysis to evaluation levels in the cognitive domain. Analysis, synthesis, and evaluation are high-end performance levels and expectations for continuing competence;

3. **Consumer Education Example**: The verbs used in the previous Consumer Education example range from knowledge to application levels in the cognitive domain. Knowledge, comprehension, and application are high-end performance levels and expectations for Consumer Education.

■ Because the learning statements are taken collectively to achieve the indicator (critical element), a sufficient number of statements must be present. Generally, four to six verb statements per indicator are desired. If there are more than ten verb statements per indicator, the indicator may contain more than one essential behavior. In this case, the indicator should be revised to address only one essential behavior. Additional indicators may be necessary.

■ The selection of terms is most important, because many terms are unclear or have multiple meanings. Using ambiguous terms like *normal*, *recognize*, or *appreciate* can have multiple meanings or interpretations, therefore, terms must be clear with common meanings or interpretations for all users.

■ All statements must be worded so performance can be measured objectively. This guideline reinforces the importance of the previous item; terms must be clear with common meanings or interpretations for all users:

  ○ **Education Example**: The learning statement in the education example given previously requires the learner to create a data collection plan that includes specified items. Although grading a project can be considered subjective, using grading rubrics will reduce subjectivity (see chapter 5 for creating rubrics);

  ○ **Continuing Competence Example**: The learning statement in the continuing competence example given previously requires the learner to interpret patient care data using a specified process and specific items to include. Once again, the use of grading rubrics will reduce subjectivity;

○ **Consumer Education Example**: The learning statement in the consumer education example given previously requires the learner to examine an insulin prescription. Many times, assessing performance of consumers is not done, but could be accomplished through questioning or a written worksheet.

■ The performance expectation for all learners is at 100% for all indicators. The indicators are the critical elements for each competency. The critical elements are the essential behaviors required for the situation, and therefore, must be demonstrated at the 100% level.

■ The performance behaviors should include only those essential for documenting competence. In identifying critical elements, it is important to separate *must perform* from *nice to know*. Although some of the nice-to-know behaviors may be included in learning experiences, only achievement of essential behaviors is measured.

Using the sample competency statements for education, continuing competence, and consumer education, example of learning statements are:

■ **Education Competency Example**: At the conclusion of the learning unit, the learner will be able to use outcome measures to evaluate effectiveness of care.

 1. Learning Statement: Data collection

   ● Create a data collection plan to include:
     ❑ A brief description of the project;
     ❑ Specific data that is needed;
     ❑ Rationale for collecting the data;
     ❑ What insight the data might provide?
     ❑ How it will help effectiveness of care?
     ❑ What will be done with the data once it has been collected?

■ **Continuing Competency Example**: At the conclusion of the learning unit, the learner will be able to use evaluative statements when charting to communicate progress toward meeting identified patient outcomes.

1. Learning Statements: Data analysis

- Interpret patient care data by:
  - ❑ Accessing patient data using facility health care information system;
  - ❑ Selecting, sorting, and summarizing patient care data;
  - ❑ Transforming patient care data into information;
  - ❑ Transforming patient care information into knowledge.

■ **Consumer Education Competency Example**: At the conclusion of the learning unit, the learner will be able to self-administer insulin using correct injection technique, site selection, and dose.

1. Learning Statements: Medication identification

- Examine insulin prescription:
  - ❑ Identify type prescribed;
  - ❑ Identify time to be administered;
  - ❑ Identify number of units prescribed.

Learning statements would need to be developed for all indicators identified within a competency statement.

EFFECTIVE METHODS FOR LEARNING COMPETENCIES

Following the general rules from Tables 4.1 and 4.2, competencies have been written and the essential behaviors needed to demonstrate each competency have been identified. The next phase in the competency-based educational process is to answer Question 3: What are the most effective ways to learn those competencies (Lenburg, 1999)? Before addressing this question, a look at learning styles is warranted.

Learning Styles

Every learner has a personal learning style, thought to be an "enduring, patterned, and preferred mode of learning" (Sproles & Sproles, 1990). Learning styles are the ways learners concentrate on, process, internal-

Table 4.2

LEARNING STATEMENTS THAT LEAD TO COMPETENT PERFORMANCE

DEVELOPING INDICATORS TO DEFINE COMPETENCIES	IDENTIFY CRITICAL ELEMENTS FOR EACH COMPETENCY
	Begin each element with a verb.
	The verb must identify the performance at the high end of the level desired.
	Four to six verb statements per critical element.
	Use terms that have common meanings or interpretations.
	Must be able to measure objectively.
	Performance expected is at 100% for all learners.
	Actions that are essential for documenting competence. Separate *must perform* from *nice to know*.

ize, and remember new and difficult information or skills (Shaughnessy, 1998). Usually, learners are not aware of their learning styles. Knowledge of learning styles is important because they influence the learning strategies selected. The selected learning strategies are influenced by the learning situation, and therefore, learners use different learning strategies (and thus, learning activities) in different learning situations (Berings, Poell, Simons, & Van Veldhoven, 2007).

There are numerous learning-style instruments available today, but most were developed for use with children in K–12 settings. The Experiential Learning Theory and its learning-style instrument, developed by Kolb (Kolb, Boyatzis, & Mainemelis, 1999), provides a multilinear model of adult development. The theory emphasizes the central role experience plays in the learning process. Following is a summary of the four basic learning styles:

Diverging: People with this learning style are best at viewing concrete situations from many different points of view. It is labeled "Diverging" because a person with it performs better in situations that call for generation of ideas, such as a "brainstorming" session. People with a Diverging learning style have broad cultural interests and like to gather information. Research shows that they are interested in people, tend to be imaginative and emotional, have broad cultural interests, and tend to specialize in the arts.

Assimilating. People with this learning style are best at understanding a wide range of information and putting it into concise, logical form. Individuals with an Assimilating style are less focused on people and more interested in ideas and abstract concepts. Generally, people with this style find it more important that a theory have logical soundness than practical value.

Converging. People with this learning style are best at finding practical uses for ideas and theories. They have the ability to solve problems and make decisions based on finding solutions to questions or problems. Individuals with a Converging learning style prefer to deal with technical tasks and problems rather than with social issues and interpersonal issues.

Accommodating. People with this learning style have the ability to learn from primarily "hands-on" experience. They enjoy carrying out plans and involving themselves in new and challenging experiences. Their tendency may be to act on "gut" feelings rather than on logical analysis. In solving problems, individuals with an Accommodating learning style rely more heavily on people for information than on their own technical analysis. (Kolb, Boyatzis, & Mainemelis, 1999, pp. 5–7)

It is generally accepted that the manner in which individuals approach a learning situation impacts performance and achievement of learning outcomes (An Update on Learning Styles/Cognitive Styles Research, 2007). Traditionally, a learner's learning style has been tested based on the use of questionnaires. However, this method has shown to be not only time-consuming, but also unreliable (Yannibelli, Godoy, & Amandi, 2006). It has also been noted that as people age their learning-style preferences become less pronounced and more variation is found among these preferences (Truluck & Courtenay, 1999). If a learner is having difficulty demonstrating competency, examine the learning strategy and learning preferences to determine if adjustments need to be made for success.

The following general guidelines outline the identification of learning activities that assist learners in achieving outstanding outcomes for each competency statement:

■ The focus must be on the desired outcomes. Never lose sight of the expected competency when selecting or designing learning activities.

○ **Education:** In traditional education, learning opportunities are usually selected by the faculty to achieve course/program objectives. Within a competency-based system, competency statements replace traditional objectives. The required competency drives the selection of learning activities.

○ **Continuing Competence:** The process for identifying competency outcomes within workplace settings is typically not as formal as it is in educational settings. Staff need direction about the behaviors expected in the employment setting; what are the expected competencies and at what performance level? Clearly communicating expectations to all staff is of utmost importance so everyone is moving in the same direction.

○ **Consumer Education:** Focusing on the expected competency with consumers is not the usual approach to patient teaching. As with continuing competence, the development and communication of patient competencies is essential if changes in health care behavior are to be achieved.

■ The content must focus on accomplishing the desired outcome. Commercially prepared learning units are abundant on the Internet (see Additional Resources) and can be used to foster learning. Many of the mass-produced learning products will contain material that is not focused specifically on the expected competency—the nice vs. the necessary. This is not a great concern because assessment of competency achievement will measure only the essential behaviors.

○ **Education Example:** *The Essentials of Baccalaureate Education for Professional Nursing Practice* (1998) delineates the content for baccalaureate programs, and competency statements must reflect that content. Additional content may surface from practice and regulation stakeholders. The newly developed competency statements should incorporate this content as long as the focus remains on the expected competency.

○ **Continuing Competence Example**: Once again, the newly developed competency statements should incorporate the addressed changes in competency requirements, work processes, or outcomes. The competencies should be used to guide content identification. Existing continuing education learning units can be used as long as the focus remains on the expected competency.

○ **Consumer Education Example**: Content selection for patient teaching is dictated by the health care issue being addressed. Specific health-related associations that support the general population may have patient teaching materials available, but the materials may not use a competency-based process. These materials can be used as long as the focus remains on the expected competency.

■ The learning method must engage learners as active participants in their own learning. Adult learning principles should be applied, as they support accountability and ownership in the learning process. Adult learning principles recommend the use of self-directed learning as a learning option whenever possible (Wright, 2005).

○ **Education Example**: The faculty typically selects learning opportunities that contribute to competency achievement, but learners also have a responsibility to identify and use additional learning activities to demonstrate their competence. By fostering learner involvement, the faculty also addresses *The Essentials of Baccalaureate Education for Professional Nursing Practice* (1998) requirement of encouraging lifelong learning.

○ **Continuing Competence Example**: The use of adult learning principles in the workplace assists in creating accountability and ownership of the competency process. Adults have a deep need to be self-directing. Staff is more accepting of the competency process if they have some control over the learning options.

○ **Consumer Education Example**: Adult learning principles also apply to consumers. First, they need to understand the importance of demonstrating competency. Why is it important to them personally? Giving consumers some control by offering options they can choose from supports active participation and is consistent with adult learning principles.

The learning method should allow for different learning styles. Disagreement exists to whether preferred learning methods are stable over time or subject to change based on past experiences and the situation. Because there is general acceptance that the manner in which individuals approach a learning situation impacts their performance and achievement of learning outcomes (*An Update on Learning Styles/ Cognitive Styles Research;* Berings, Poell, Simons, & Van Veldhoven, 2007), providing a variety of learning methods allows for learners to choose the method that fits their preferred learning style the closest.

Using Kolb's (Kolb, Boyatzis, & Mainemelis, 1999) four basic learning styles, the following summarizes the preferred learning method:

Diverging: In formal learning situations, people with the Diverging style prefer to work in groups, listening with an open mind and receiving personalized feedback.

Assimilating. In formal learning situations, people with this style prefer readings, lectures, exploring analytical models, and having time to think things through.

Converging. In formal learning situations, people with this style prefer to experiment with new ideas, simulations, laboratory assignments, and practical applications.

Accommodating. In formal learning situations, people with the Accommodating learning style prefer to work with others to get assignments done, to set goals, to do field work, and to test out different approaches to completing a project. (Kolb, Boyatzis, & Mainemelis, 1999, pp. 5–7)

○ **Education Example**: In many traditional educational programs, preferred teaching style seems to predominate. The learner is forced to adapt his or her preferred learning style to the particular faculty's teaching style. Although faculty knows about different learning styles, teaching methods do not reflect application of this knowledge. Actual practice supports the delivery of large amounts of content in a limited amount of time to a large group of learners, a one-size-fits-all approach. Developing a variety of learning activities leading to the same desired outcome would allow learners to select the activity best suited to their learning preference.

○ **Continuing Competence Example**: The learning-style instruments commonly used in educational settings should not automatically be used in the workplace because they do not address the social learning dimension; they focus on the ways that learners process information offered by teachers and textbooks, and they limit the learners' responses to those of formal learning situations (Berings, Poell, Simons, & Van Veldhoven, 2007). Berings et al. have developed an on-the-job learning styles questionnaire for the nursing profession. They contend it describes nurses learning styles by providing a profile of the different learning activities that nurses use in different learning situations.

○ **Consumer Education Example**: Consumer learning and decision-making styles are different measures, but the two can be helpful in understanding how consumers learn and why they choose to engage in learning activities (Sproles & Sproles, 1990). With the aging population and the resultant need to manage chronic illnesses, understanding how and why older adults seek learning situations is essential for patient educators. It is suggested that not all older learners are active, hands-on learners as adult education literature suggests, but rather with age there is a tendency to become more reflective and observational in the learning environment (Truluck & Courtenay, 1999).

Learning methods should use realistic strategies (problem-based learning, case studies, simulations, team projects, etc.) and align with real-world situations (see Table 4.3). There are many commercially prepared learning units available online (see Additional Resources). Most are designed for independent study and include an objective test at the end of the learning unit. In many cases, the learning units are free but there is a fee for the examination. Because the focus of competency outcomes is on *doing*, not on *knowing* or *knowing how to do*, using the learning unit's examination as a measure of competency is insufficient for demonstrating competency. The commercial products would need to be revised to be performance-based, or some form of performance-based assessment that requires the application of the presented materials to real-world situations would be necessary. The focus of the learning activities must be on demonstration of desired outcomes, not on the input and process the learner uses to achieve the desired outcomes.

○ **Education**: Too often lecture is the primary teaching method employed in traditional higher education programs. Lecturing fosters passive learning and passive learners. With a competency-based system, learners must be active participants in their learning. Simulations, clinical experiences, and problem-based learning are learning strategies that require the learner to be an active participant in achieving expected outcomes. With the change to making learners accountable for their learning, the faculty role as provider of all information changes to one of facilitator, guiding the learner to actually perform to competency expectations. Most of the current traditional learning activities would need to be repurposed to performance-based activities.

○ **Continuing Competence**: In the work setting, staff is responsible and accountable for being competent practitioners. The organization will define expected competencies based upon internal and external demands. In many cases, staff is allowed to choose the learning method they will use to meet the expected competencies. This flexibility reinforces personal responsibility and accountability for maintaining competence and promotes active learning. Unlike traditional educational situations, social learning processes may be used in the workplace to gain competence. With social learning, people learn from one another through observational learning, imitation, and modeling.

○ **Consumer Education**: Patient education adds value to the management of personal health, and specific interventions aimed at improving patient knowledge and skills can improve health outcomes. Many health providers provide written materials to patients so they can self-educate on their own time. In addition, many consumers search the Internet for information about health conditions, sometimes with questionable results. The abundance and variety of educa-

Table 4.3

EFFECTIVE METHODS FOR LEARNING COMPETENCIES	
Identifying learning activities	The focus must be on the desired outcomes. Never lose sight of the expected competency.
	The content must focus on accomplishing the desired outcome.
	The learning method must engage the learner as an active participant in his/her own learning.
	The learning method should allow for different learning styles.
	Learning methods should use realistic strategies (problem-based learning, case studies, simulations, team projects, etc.).

tional materials can be overwhelming to most learners. Although printed and nonprinted materials are important tangible supplements, they may not meet the consumers' needs, or help move them toward competency achievement. Reading printed material is not *doing*. Medline Plus (2008) does offer interactive consumer education materials (see Additional Resources). With most of the patient-education materials available, there needs to be one more step in the competency process, and that's where the consumer takes action to become competent.

DECISIONS ABOUT MEASURING COMPETENCY

Lenburg's fourth and last question, "What are the most effective ways to document that learners and/or practitioners have achieved the required competencies?" (1999, p. 3) focuses on performance-assessment methods to provide evidence that competency expectations have been met.

Assessments should measure more than knowledge. They must measure integration of knowledge in real-world situations. Performance

Table 4.4

DECISIONS ABOUT MEASURING COMPETENCY	
Creating competency performance assessments	Assessments measure more than knowledge. They must measure integration of knowledge in real-world situations.
	Assessments are criterion-referenced.
	Assessments are summative, not formative.
	Assessments are comparable across learners.
	Assessments are administered consistently across testing situations.
	A variety of assessment types is used.
	Assessment expectations are that 100% of the learners demonstrate competency of the essential behaviors desired.
	Assessments are graded in an objective manner.

assessments must correspond with the competencies to be assessed (see Table 4.4).

According to the COPA model (Lenburg, 1999), competency assessments should be criterion-referenced because learners' performance is compared with a set of expected behaviors, the competency statements:

- Assessments should be summative, although formative evaluations can be used in the interim to assist the learner in identifying areas where additional study is needed;
- Assessments must be comparable across learners. Different learners at different times should be assessed at the same level of difficulty with the same competency requirements;
- Assessments should be administered consistently across testing situations. Evaluators should administer the assessment in the same manner to all learners at all times in all situations;
- Comprehensive assessment of competencies should use a variety of assessment types: simulation, actual performance, and written examinations. Ideally, alternate forms of assessments should be

available. Alternate forms must be comparable in level of difficulty and competency expectations;

■ Competency-based learning requires that the identified essential competencies be performed completely by all learners. Decisions will need to be made about how many times a learner will be allowed to retest. There also must be a process where the learner is informed about areas below standards so remediation can occur;

■ Assessment evaluators must use the same grading protocols to maximize interrater reliability. The goal is to have all assessments graded in an objective manner, using established grading protocols. Subjective grading should not be an issue.

Chapter 5 presents detailed information about creating performance assessments to measure competence.

■ **Education Example:** Creating objective performance assessments can be challenging and time-consuming for faculty. A comprehensive assessment plan that measures the essential outcomes needs to be developed. Objective performance assessments require a change in beliefs about assessment types and purpose. Decisions about the types of assessments to use that best measure the essential competencies must be made. Although knowledge is important, the integration of knowledge into real practice situations should guide assessment development.

The process for determining a grade can also be challenging because higher education institutions have grading policies that may not allow for competency-based assessment processes. Whereas most institutions are required by regional accrediting agencies to report specified outcomes, the change to outcome-based courses/programs may be supported by administration.

Lenburg (1999) stresses that there is a time for learning and a time for testing, and that the two times should not be confused. Faculty roles during the learning process are those of mentor or facilitator, but once the assessment process begins, faculty roles change to those of evaluator. Learners must be able to clearly distinguish between the learning period and the testing period. Faculty should not maintain a running summary of events during the learning period to be used as the summative evaluation at the end of the learning period. Any formative evaluation is to be used to help a learner identify where additional work is required.

■ **Continuing Competence**: Wright (2005) has developed sample worksheets for tracking staff competency achievement (see Additional Resources). The responsibility of demonstrating competency and providing the documentation rests with the individual employee. The evidence required to support achievement of expected competencies is similar to a portfolio. Each employee must provide documentation in a predefined form. Employees could also be asked about their personal/professional development and improvement (Berings et al., 2007). Many times, employees gain competence in areas other than the ones identified by the organization. Wright also provides worksheets to assist with performance appraisals and annual evaluations.

■ **Consumer Education**: Performance evaluation of consumer knowledge and skill integration is more difficult because a formal evaluation process usually doesn't exist. Evaluation is typically based on how well chronic conditions are managed or how often the consumer re-enters the health care system. Even if a formal evaluation system exists, once the consumer leaves the provider, performance of required competencies depends on whether the consumer chooses to adhere to expectations. The challenge is to make the consumer want to change personal behavior.

SUMMARY

Using Lenburg's (1999) COPA model, changing to a competency-based method can be accomplished. The model uses four basis questions to guide the change to a competency-based process. The process entails the identification of essential behaviors and converting the essential behaviors into competency statements. The competency statements are written to require the learner to *do*, not just *know* or *know how to do* a required behavior. Once the competency statements have been written, learning statements are developed to correspond to each competency statement. Learning statements are based on indicators, critical behaviors necessary to meet the competency. The next step requires the identification of learning activities that support each indicator. Learning activities should require the learner to perform the specified behavior,

Exhibit 4.1

ESSENTIAL QUESTIONS	RESPONSES TO QUESTIONS
1. What are the essential competencies and outcomes for contemporary practice in your setting?	
2. What are the indicators (critical elements) that define the competencies for your setting?	
3. What are the most effective methods for learning the identified competencies?	
4. What are the most effective ways to document that learners and/or practitioners have achieved the required competencies?	

CONSUMER COMPETENCE ACTIVITY ESSENTIAL QUESTIONS	RESPONSES TO QUESTIONS
1. What are the essential competencies and outcomes for consumer competence?	
2. What are the indicators (critical elements) that define the expected competencies for the consumer?	
3. What are the most effective methods for consumers to learn the identified competencies?	
4. What are the most effective ways to document that consumers have achieved the required competencies?	

From Lenburg (1999).

thus, the learner must be an active participant in the learning process. Learning activities should be varied and incorporate the preferred learning style of the learner. Decisions need to be made about how competency will be measured. Using a combination of objective and performance measures is recommended. Assessments should be criterion-referenced and summative in nature. The expectation for learners is 100% achievement of the desired essential competencies. Unsuccessful learners should have the opportunity to repeat an assessment after appropriate remediation.

CHAPTER 4 ACTIVITY

Chapters 1, 2, and 3 provided a foundation for developing a competency-based education (CBE) program or course and how to use the COPA model. This chapter applied the COPA model to higher education, continuing competence, and consumer education. Review your activities from the three previous chapters. Depending on your setting and goals, answer Lenburg's four questions to further develop your CBE program or course. Exhibit 4.1 offers you the opportunity to answer the competency questions posed in this chapter yourself.

REFERENCES

Adams Center for Teaching Excellence. (2005). *Learning taxonomies*. Retrieved August 8, 2009, from
http://www.acu.edu/academics/adamscenter/resources/coursedev/t axonomies.html
Alspach, G. (2008). Recognizing the primacy of competency and exposing the existence of incompetence. *Critical Care Nurse, 28*(4), 12–14.
American Association of Colleges of Nursing. (1998). *The essentials of baccalaureate education for professional nursing practice*. Washington, DC: Author.
Berings, M., Poell, R., Simons, P., & Van Veldhoven, M. (2007). The development and validation of the on-the-job learning styles questionnaire for the nursing profession. *Journal of Advanced Nursing, 58*(5), 480–492.
Dooley, K., & Lindner, J. (2002). Competency-based behavioral anchors as authentication tools to document distance education competencies. *Journal of Agricultural Education, 43*(1), 24–35.
The Joint Commission. (2005). *Comprehensive accreditation manual for hospitals: The official handbook*. Oakbrook Terrance, IL: Joint Commission Resources.
Kolb, D. A., Boyatzis, R. E., & Mainemelis, C. (1999). *Experiential learning theory: Previous research and new directions*. Department of Organizational Behavior, Weath-

erhead School of Management, Case Western Reserve University. Retrieved August 8, 2009, from http://www.medizin1.klinikum.uni-erlangen.de/e113/e191/e1223/e1228/e989/inhalt990/erfahrungslernen _2004_ger.pdf

Lenburg, C. B. (1999). The framework, concepts, and methods of the competency outcomes and performance assessment (COPA) model. *Online Journal of Issues in Nursing, 4*(3). Retrieved December 15, 2008, from http://www.nursingworld.org/ojin

Meretoja, R., Isoaho, H., & Leino-Kilpi, H. (2004, July 15). Nurse competence scale: Development and psychometric testing. *Journal of Advanced Nursing, 47*(2), 124–133.

O'Shea, K. (2002). *Staff development nursing secrets: Questions and answers reveal the secrets to successful staff development.* Philadelphia: Hanley & Belfus.

Redfern, S., Norman, I., Calman, L., Watson, R., & Murrells, T. (2002). Assessing competence to practice in nursing: A review of the literature. *Research Papers in Education, 17*(1), 51–77.

Redman, R. W., Lenburg, C. B., & Hinton-Walker, P. (1999). Competency assessment: Methods for development and evaluation in nursing education. *Online Journal of Issues in Nursing, 4*(3). Retrieved December 15, 2008, from http://www.nursingworld.org/ojin

Sadler-Smith, E., & Smith, P. (2004, July). Strategies for accommodating individuals' styles and preferences in flexible learning programmes. *British Journal of Educational Technology, 35*(4), 395–412.

Shaughnessy, M. (1998). An interview with Rita Dunn about learning styles. *Clearing House, 71*(3), 141.

Sproles, E., & Sproles, G. (1990). Consumer decision-making styles as a function of individual learning styles. *Journal of Consumer Affairs, 24*(1), 134–147.

Truluck, J., & Courtenay, B. (1999, April). Learning style preferences among older adults. *Educational Gerontology, 25*(3), 221–236.

Whelan, L. (2006). Competency assessment of nursing staff. *Orthopaedic Nursing, 25*(3), 198.

Wright, D. (2005). *The ultimate guide to competency assessment in health care* (3rd ed.). Minneapolis, MN: Creative Health Care Management.

Yannibelli, V., Godoy, D., & Amandi, A. (2006, April). A genetic algorithm approach to recognise students' learning styles. *Interactive Learning Environments, 14*(1), 55–78.

ADDITIONAL RESOURCES

Consumer Education

Harvard Medical School (2009). Pri-Med Patient Education Center. *http://www.patient educationcenter.org/*

JAMA Patient Page. *http://jama.ama-assn.org/cgi/collection/patient_page*

Medline Plus (August 2008). Interactive Health Tutorials. *http://www.nlm.nih.gov/medlineplus/tutorial.html*

Ohio State University Medical Center (2009). Patient education materials. *http://medicalcenter.osu.edu/patientcare/patient_education/Pages/index.aspx*

University of California, San Francisco (n.d.). *http://www.ucsfhealth.org/adult/health_library/patient_educati on.html*
University of Pittsburg Medical Center (2009). UPMC Patient Education Materials. *http://www.upmc.com/healthAtoZ/patienteducation/Pages/patiented.aspx*

Nursing Continuing Education

AHC Media *http://www.freecme.com/gcourses1.php?sub=byspecialty*
ANA Online Continuing Education *http://nursingworld.org/CE/cehome.cfm*

- College @ Home *http://www.collegeathome.com/open-courseware/health-medical/nursing/*
- Medi-Smart *http://www.medi-smart.com/freeceu.htm*
- Medscape *http://www.medscape.com/viewarticle/412274*
- MyFreeCE *http://www.myfreece.com/welcome.asp?source=google 2&term=contin uing+education+nursing*
- Nursing Spectrum *http://www.nurse.com/ce/*
- RnCeus.com *http://www.rnceus.com/*
- rn.com *http://www.rn.com/main.php?uniq=88717&command= manage_courselis t&data[submit_value]=Course%20Catalog*
- rn.org *http://www.rn.org/CourseCatalog.php*

Worksheets for Changing to A Competency-Based System

Wright, D. (2005a). Worksheet for identifying ongoing competencies *http://www.chcm.com/docs/compwks_ongoing.pdf*
Wright, D. (2005b). Competency assessment worksheet *http://www.chcm.com/docs/compwks_assmt.pdf*
Wright, D. (2005c). Supervisor summary of employee competency completion worksheet *http://www.chcm.com/docs/compswks_empcomp.pdf*
Wright, D. (2005d). Supervisor evaluation of overall competency completion *http://www.chcm.com/docs/compwks_ovrleval.pdf*

5

Developing Valid and Reliable Assessments

JANICE L. McCOY
MARION G. ANEMA

OVERVIEW

This chapter reviews reliability and validity processes to help ensure high-quality assessment tools. Assessment development that reflects each learning statement and the typical learner domains (cognitive, affective, and psychomotor) is addressed, including the need for adequate preparation and the expertise of item writers and reviewers. The steps in developing objective and performance assessments are explored. Standard setting for assessments is explained, and several standard-setting methods are presented.

INTRODUCTION

Once competency statements are written, a process to assess competency must be developed. The competency statements tell us what performance is expected and guide the selection of the assessment method most likely to provide the desired results. In order to achieve outstanding outcomes, assessments must be valid and reliable. Close attention to validity and reliability increases confidence in the assessment method and the actual assessment results.

VALIDITY AND RELIABILITY

With the focus on achieving outstanding outcomes, assessment development is of paramount importance. Educators must facilitate independent learning, encourage the development of critical thinking and evaluate learning (Snelgrove & Slater, 2003). At the same time, educators must meet the demands of multiple stakeholders: higher education institutions, regulatory agencies, employers, and consumers. Poorly constructed assessments cannot accurately measure desired outcomes, thus assessment developers must create valid and reliable assessments in order to achieve outstanding outcomes.

Validity

Validity of an assessment is indispensable, and no quality or virtue of an assessment can compensate for inadequate validity. The most simplistic definition of validity is the degree to which an assessment measures what it is supposed to measure, and that it is valid for a particular purpose and for a particular group. Validation efforts typically focus on what exactly is measured by an assessment and whether what is measured corresponds to the theoretical domain(s) originally specified (Hill, Dean, & Goffney, 2007). In competency-based education, assessments must correspond to and measure the stated competency.

The attributes of validity are relevance, accuracy, and utility (Billings & Halstead, 2005). Assessments that are relevant must directly measure the competency and/or the learning statement. Assessments are accurate if they precisely measure the competency and/or the learning statement. Assessments have utility if the assessment results can be used for evaluation and improvement (Billings & Halstead).

Assessments are designed for a variety of purposes, and validity can be evaluated only in terms of a purpose. Although there are several different types of validity, all are under the broad area of measurement validity. Billings and Halstead (2005) list three categories within measurement validity: content, criterion, and construct validity. For maximum support, it is ideal to have data from each of the three categories.

■ **Content validity** provides evidence that the assessment samples relevant content. Educators, current practice demands, and professional standards of practice define relevant content. An example is an assessment that addresses all content presented in a course or program.

■ **Criterion validity** provides evidence that the assessment measures current and future performance. Results from standardized assessments used for certification or licensing are often used as a comparison. For example, there is a positive relationship between program scores and certification or licensing scores.

■ **Construct validity** provides evidence that the assessment shows a relationship between performance on the assessment and some attribute to be measured. The competency statements should describe the desired attributes clearly. An example is the relationship between learner attributes, such as IQ or previous experience, and program/course outcomes.

Reliability

Closely related to the concept of validity is the concept of reliability. Reliability is the degree to which an assessment consistently measures what it says it will measure. Validity findings can be in jeopardy if an assessment is unreliable. Like validity, there are categories of reliability: stability, equivalence, and internal consistency (Billings & Halstead, 2005).

■ **Stability reliability** is the consistency of an assessment over time. Will assessment scores be consistent for different groups of learners?

■ **Equivalence reliability** is the degree to which two different forms of the assessment will produce the same results. Is there a difference in scores whether Form A or Form B of an assessment is used?

■ **Internal consistency reliability** is the extent to which all items on an assessment measure the same variable. Internal consistency reliability is only used when the assessment is measuring just one concept at a time.

Unfortunately, no assessment is perfectly reliable. The reliability of assessments can be improved by increasing the number of items on the assessment, or by using group results rather than individual student results. For objective assessments, the general rule is one test item per minute for moderately difficult multiple-choice items (Billings & Halstead, 2005). The number of assessment items affects reliability, thus increasing the number of items will increase reliability.

When scoring assessments, such as psychomotor skill demonstration, essays, research papers, and so on, involves subjectivity, there are concerns with interrater reliability and/or intrarater reliability. Interrater reliability concentrates on the reliability of two or more independent scorers. Intrarater reliability focuses on the reliability of individual scorers. Scoring and rating are sources of errors of measurement; therefore, if multiple scorers are used, it is important to estimate the consistency of the scorers' ratings. This can be accomplished by having all scorers rate the same assessment and calculate the percentage of agreements/disagreements of the scorers. Using rubrics as a scoring guide can also increase interrater reliability.

ASSESSMENT DEVELOPMENT

Assessments are designed for a variety of purposes. The purpose of the assessment will guide the type of assessment selected. Validity of an assessment is also dependent on the stated purpose of the assessment; therefore, the assessment type must be appropriate for the learning domain (cognitive, affective, psychomotor) and the desired competency or learning statement.

Writing Learning Statements

Each identified competency is supported by detailed learning statements. Learning statements are similar to the traditional objectives, in that they address:

- One of the learning domains (cognitive, affective, or psychomotor);
- Measurement of one behavior;
- Action verbs used to determine complexity of the task;
- Learner-focused orientation.

Learning statements differ from most traditional objectives in that they:

- Support a desired competency;
- Require demonstration of competency for every learning statement;
- Are practice driven rather than course-content driven.

Learning statements are the foundation for creating assessments. It is of paramount importance that assessment items align with every learning statement. In competency-based learning, demonstration of competency is required for all learning statements. Learning statements will also determine the assessment method selected. A variety of assessment methods must be considered. Knowing how to perform is not the same as actually performing; therefore, objective-based and performance-based assessment methods must be employed.

OBJECTIVE-BASED ASSESSMENTS

Many health care fields are practice disciplines that require application and synthesis of previously acquired knowledge, skills, and attitudes. Reading and answering multiple-choice questions are not activities required in professional practice. Hill, Dean, and Goffney (2007) allege that multiple-choice assessments focus narrowly on basic skills and do not measure learners' abilities to solve complex, real-world problems. Therefore, there may be a disconnect between an assessment domain and the knowledge, skills, and practice domains that are to be measured by an assessment.

For this reason, objective-based assessments cannot be the only assessment method employed. Objective-based assessments are appropriate when a competency requires learners to *know* information or *know how* to perform a skill or apply information in a given situation. Care must be taken to develop assessment items at the application level, rather than at the lower cognitive learning domains. Assessment items must align with the competency and learning statements previously developed (see chapter 4).

Preparation of Item Writers for Objective Assessments

The quality and relevance of objective assessments depends on the expertise of item writers. In addition, content validity will depend on the quality of the assessment items, which, in turn, is dependent on the qualifications of the item writers. Having a mix of educators, employers, and professional standards personnel, knowledgeable about current practice standards, is essential. Preparation of item writers is crucial for development of appropriate objective-based items.

Instructional sessions should precede actual item writing. Item writers should understand the purpose and the process to be used in creating assessment items. Providing copies of all competencies and learning statements will help item writers understand the task at hand. The item-writing task requires assessment items that align with the competencies and learning statements; therefore, item writers must clearly understand what the desired competencies are so items can be written to the appropriate difficulty level. Reviewing the desired competencies and the supporting learning statements with item writers will focus the item writing on the desired outcomes. This review also functions as further validation by content experts of the appropriateness of the competency/learning statements. Another benefit of reviewing the statements with the assessment item writers is to validate the chosen assessment method (objective or performance).

Instruction on constructing objective assessment items should occur so items measure what they are supposed to measure. Whether assessment items are matching, ordering, or multiple choice, assessment items must follow the same basic format. The person responsible for the assessment development and item-writing session will determine the structure and format of assessment items beforehand and communicate this information to item writers. Table 5.1 presents a checklist of the areas to cover with item writers.

In a multiple-choice item, similarity and plausibility of response options represent primary factors contributing to the difficulty or easiness of the item. Multiple-choice items should align with the level of difficulty expected. Assessment items can be written at the knowledge, comprehension, application, or analysis level of Bloom's taxonomy (Forehand, 2008). Each assessment item must have an appropriate number of response options. Four or more answer options are recommended, but the number should not exceed eight options. It is never acceptable to use options such as *All of the Above, None of the Above, A and B*, and so on. The goal is to control the guessing factor. The acceptable minimum standard for guessing is 0.25 (Voorhees, 2001).

Table 5.1

ITEM-WRITING CHECKLIST

1. Review competency/learning statements with item writers.
2. Either assign learning statements for item development to writers or allow them to self-select statements based on their expertise.
3. Develop a question stem that aligns with the assigned learning statement and focuses on one thought, problem, or idea. Try to keep the stems short.
4. All information needed to answer the question must be present but must not provide clues to the correct answer.
5. Create clear and plausible answers to the question. The guessing factor should be 0.25 or less.
6. Write items to the appropriate difficulty level.
7. If an item calls for a judgment, include the criteria for making that judgment.
8. Avoid:

   ■ Words that are overly complex or have multiple meanings;
   ■ Using "NOT" in the stem;
   ■ Absolute and imprecise modifiers;
   ■ Localization or sensitivity issues.

9. Items should be readable and obey all the rules of grammar and usage.

Items must be defensible; therefore, item writers must have current resources to support correct answers for each assessment item. It is not acceptable to support correct answers by saying it is common knowledge or because this is the way it's always been done.

Standard Setting

Seventy percent (70%) is often the standard passing score, the minimum established competency level, for many throughout their educational experience. If higher performance levels are desired, then the minimum passing score needs to reflect this higher expectation. An example is dosage calculation competency. Setting 70% as a minimum passing score is not acceptable. One hundred percent on a calculation assessment may be the desired outcome, but is it realistic? The minimum acceptable passing score for dosage calculations must be determined. Standard setting is a method of determining the cut score or the passing score corresponding to the desired performance level. One approach to setting an absolute performance standard is referred to as the criterion-referenced method, and involves linking decisions about assessment performance to criteria for acceptable practice of the relevant profession.

The competency and learning statements are the criteria used to identify acceptable practice. The purpose is to set a performance standard on the assessment with the expectation that those who meet the standard will be judged competent in practice, and those who are not judged competent in practice will fail the assessment and be referred for remediation so they can meet the minimum competency standard.

Determining the minimum level of competence required for a learning situation can be a difficult task. The adequacy of a standard-setting method depends on two processes:

- Whether the judges adequately conceptualize the (minimum) competency of target examinees;
- Whether judges adequately estimate item difficulty based on their conceptualized examinee competency.

Two popular methods used to determine cut scores are the Angoff method and the Bookmark method.

Angoff Method

The Angoff method is the oldest and most-researched method used (Voorhees, 2001). The Angoff method is frequently used to set standards on high-stakes multiple-choice educational, licensure, and credentialing examinations. The Angoff method attempts to establish valid, meaningful cut scores (minimum passing score).

In a standard-setting work session, a group of expert judges considers the meaning of a just-minimally-competent or just-qualified examinee. This group of 12 or more contributes to assessment validity. The judges are asked to estimate the proportion of a borderline group that would answer each item on the assessment correctly. The estimated performance standard for each judge is determined by summing the item judgments. The resulting Angoff rating is aggregated for all of the judges. This aggregated score is then used as a performance standard (cut score) for the assessment.

Preparation and Expertise of Item Judges. Selection and training of item judges is a critical aspect of any standard-setting process, and the Angoff process is no exception. Having a mix of educators, employers, and personnel knowledgeable about current practice standards is essential. In addition, the concept of a minimally competent professional is the key to successful implementation of the Angoff method. Various names are given to this hypothetical person, including *just-qualified candidate* and *minimally acceptable candidate*. Regardless of the terminology used, this just-qualified examinee is a hypothetical individual who would just barely perform to expectations.

Standard-setting judges are asked to focus their attention on the individual who just meets the minimum requirements, rather than on the average, ideal, or top professional. The goal is to create a common understanding among experts about the competencies and achievement characteristics of the target examinee (Giraud, Impara, & Plake, 2005). Throughout the Angoff process, the judges must be reminded not to overestimate the just-qualified examinee's ability. A great deal of time and care must be taken to train the judges on the concept of a just-qualified professional and on the knowledge, skills, and abilities of that just-qualified individual.

Before the actual rating begins, the judges are shown several multiple-choice items without answers. The judges are asked to review these practice items and estimate the probability of a just-qualified examinee answering each item correctly. Judges assign a percentage of just-qualified examinees that would answer the item correctly, based on a hypothetical group of 100 just-qualified examinees. For example, if a judge believes that half of the just-qualified examinees would answer the item correctly, the rating would be 0.50 or 50% for that item.

After rating the practice items, the judges are given the correct answers and allowed to modify their rating if they think an adjustment is appropriate. There may be situations where a judge rates an item either very high (95%) or very low (20%). The extreme ratings are referred to as *outliers*. If outliers occur, the judge is asked whether reasons exist for the high or low rating, i.e., misunderstood the question or choices, or clarification of the definition of the just-qualified examinee.

The results of each judge are shown, and the judges are then given another opportunity to change their rating. Using a previously administered assessment for the practice session allows the use of past assessment results for comparison with the judges' rating.

Item judges' subject-matter knowledge can impact the setting of standard cut scores. Judges tend to set high standards for items they can answer correctly, and low standards for items they answer incorrectly (Verheggen, Muijtiens, and Van Os, 2008). It is important to frequently review the description of the just-qualified examinee with the item judges to minimize standard cut score errors.

After reviewing the results for the practice items, the judges continue to rate the actual items on the assessment. Following the same procedures used for the practice items, answers are given after the initial round of item rating and judges are allowed to reconsider their ratings. After the final results are compiled, the average of all ratings is calculated; this average represents the recommended cut score or performance standard that an examinee must achieve in order to pass the assessment.

The goal is to set a standard high enough so that it reliably distinguishes between those who are competent and those who are not, but not so high that the standard excludes those who are competent from meeting the standard. The validity of the assessment depends on the validity of this standard. The advantages of the Angoff method are:

■ The Angoff method of standard setting focuses the judges on what is actually expected of a successful examinee. In other words, the standard on the assessment is determined by what is expected in practice. This is considered the greatest advantage;

■ The Angoff approach allows the judges to see the entire assessment as a whole, as the examinee sees it, rather than just one question at a time;

■ Seeing all the questions allows the judges to form a more realistic perception of the relative difficulty of individual questions within the context of that assessment.

Although there are several advantages to the Angoff method, there are also challenges:

■ The greatest challenge in the Angoff process involves keeping the judges' focus on the likely performance of the just-qualified examinee. Often judges will state that the just-qualified examinee *should* answer this question correctly. The proper focus is not on what the just-qualified examinees *should* do, but what they *will* do. Judges need

Table 5.2

ANGOFF PROCESS

1. Prepare a clear and concise definition of the just-qualified examinee.
2. Gather a group of content experts for a rating session.
3. Review the definition of just-qualified examinee. Each judge must fully understand this definition.
4. Using practice items without answers, have each judge assign what percentage of 100 just-qualified examinees would answer each item correctly. No discussion should occur at this step.
5. Judges are given the correct answers and allowed to change their ratings, if appropriate.
6. Judges are provided with the ratings of all judges and discuss items with large rating ranges. Changes can be made if warranted. Remember that level of expertise in the content area will impact the judges' ratings.
7. Percentages for each judge are averaged and then the group average is calculated. The result will represent the cut score (minimum passing score) for the assessment.
8. If the practice items have been used in previous testing situations, compare the previous assessment results with the judge's results.
9. Once the item judges are comfortable with the process using practice items, repeat steps 3–6 for the new assessment.

---

to be reminded that the just-qualified examine is not necessarily the person that they would want to hire or work with. Rather, the just-qualified candidate is someone who has minimal competency;

■ The Angoff process has been criticized as setting minimum standards when higher standards may be preferred or necessary for safe practice. Minimally prepared examinees may not be able to meet the real-world expectations of employers and consumers;

■ Another challenge is resisting the tendency on the part of the judges to revert to the mean. The outlier judges may have seen something in the question that made their rating legitimate, and ample time must be allotted to discuss this. The standard-setting processes must be conducive to discussion of these outliers, but discipline has had to be exercised to resist the tendency to silently accept the majority estimate as being correct. Adequate time and discussion must be planned into the process;

■ Yet another challenge has been the fatigue factor on the part of the judges, who need to maintain focus equally on each question throughout the rating process. Adequate break time must be scheduled to mitigate fatigue and enable the judges to maintain their concentration. Table 5.2 summarizes the Angoff process.

Bookmark Method

The Bookmark standard-setting procedure was developed to address the perceived problems with the Angoff method for setting cut scores. Like Angoff, the Bookmark standard-setting procedure is a research-based method that is used by committees of educators to establish cut scores on assessments. The Bookmark procedure is based on item-response theory, a framework that characterizes the proficiency of examinees and the difficulty of test items simultaneously (Lin, n.d.).

The main difference between the two approaches is that in Angoff, judges have to assign probabilities for borderline examinees answering each item correctly, whereas in Bookmark, items are presented to judges in ascending difficulty order, and they merely have to judge the most difficult item that a borderline examinee would pass with a given probability (Schagen & Bragshaw, 2003). For the Bookmark procedure, the specified probability of success is set to 0.67 (Lin, n.d.).

Preparation and Expertise of Item Judges. Like the Angoff process, judges are selected based on their expertise in the content and practice domains. The minimum number of judges suggested is 18, but 24 judges is recommended. Typically, the judges are divided into three or four small groups to allow for greater discussion among participants. Each group consists of five to seven members.

Group leaders are identified, and the standard-setting schedule and specific leadership responsibilities are reviewed. Group leaders must be able to facilitate group discussion, keep the group focused on the task, and stay within the time allotted. During the training session for judges, a brief review is provided on the:

- Purpose of the assessment;
- Content standards;
- General and/or specific performance-level descriptions;
- Stakes associated with the assessment and the performance levels.

There are three rating rounds to the Bookmark procedure. During Round One, judges become familiar with the ordered item booklet, set initial bookmarks, and then discuss the placements. In this round, judges working in their small groups discuss what each item measures and what makes an item more difficult than the preceding item. The general performance descriptors for basic, proficient, and advanced performance levels are presented and discussed. Judges are asked to discuss and determine the content that examinees should master for placement in a given performance level.

Each judge independently determines or bookmarks a cut point. One bookmark is placed for basic, proficient, and advanced levels. Items preceding the judge's bookmark reflects content that all examinees at the given performance level are expected to know and be able to perform successfully with a probability of at least 0.67.

Round Two involves having each judge place bookmarks corresponding to the placements of other judges. For example, a group of six people would result in each judge having six bookmarks for each cut point. Differences are discussed and each judge is allowed to make changes to his or her cut points. The median of the Round Two bookmarks for each cut point is taken as that group's recommendation for that cut point.

Round Three begins with the presentation of impact data to the large group. The percentage of examinees falling into each performance level is presented, based on each group's median cut score from Round Two. With this information on how examinees actually performed, the judges discuss the bookmarks in the large group and then independently make their Round Three judgments of where to place the bookmarks. The median for the large group is considered to be the final cut point for a given performance level.

Based on the final cut scores set, performance-level descriptors are then written by the judges. Performance descriptors describe the specific knowledge, skills, and abilities held by examinees at a given performance level. Items prior to the bookmark(s) reflect the content that examinees at this performance level (basic, proficient, and advanced) are expected to answer correctly with at least a 0.67 likelihood (Schagen & Bragshaw, 2003).

Advantages of the Bookmark method are:

■ Judges have to make fewer, more tightly focused, decisions, thus reducing cognitive complexity. Judges are asked to determine what evidence is needed to satisfy the definition of competence;

- The definition of a hypothetical, just-qualified examinee is not necessary;
- Bookmark accommodates constructed-response as well as objective-based assessment items;
- Bookmark efficiently accommodates multiple cut scores at the basic, proficient, and advanced levels;
- Bookmark accommodates multiple test forms in one standard setting.

Although there are several advantages to the Bookmark Method, there are also several challenges:

- The item-ordering process can be complex, requiring computer programs to complete the task;
- With Bookmark, items are ordered according to a correct response probability of 0.67. Using a correct response probability other than 0.67 could result in items being ordered differently;
- Disagreement among judges on ordering the items is an issue in virtually all applications of the Bookmark method;
- The ordering of items from easy to difficult is considered an advantage, because it reduces the cognitive requirement on the

Table 5.3

BOOKMARK PROCESS

1. Assessment items are ordered from easy to difficult.
2. Gather a group of content experts for a rating session.
3. In Round One rating, ordered items are discussed related to what the item measures and why the item is more difficult than previous items.
4. Individually, judges identify the initial point in the ordered list of items where an examinee knew the correct answer to all items below this point.
5. In Round Two, ratings of all judges are shared and differences are discussed. Following the discussion, judges provide a second rating.
6. In Round Three, the median rating for all judges is shared and impact data are provided about the number of examinee failures if the median rating was used as the cut score.
7. The impact of using the median score is discussed and individual judges are given the opportunity to make a third rating.
8. The overall median from Round Three is used to generate the recommended passing score.

part of the judges. This ordering can be a disadvantage because it does not allow judges to relate the importance of items above or below the bookmark to curricular relevance or job performance requirements. Table 5.3 summarizes the Bookmark process.

Objective assessments have an important part in assessing competency, but cannot address the range of behaviors needed to verify competency. The next sections focus on performance-based assessments.

PERFORMANCE-BASED ASSESSMENTS

As described earlier, objective assessments have limitations, especially in practice disciplines. Because competency-based education (CBE) focuses on learners' ability to *do*, relying solely on objective assessment methods is inappropriate. Performance assessments are appropriate for measuring skills and higher level cognitive reasoning.

Performance-based assessments are commonly associated with psychomotor skills. For example, demonstrating competency in taking vital signs and carrying out direct care activities are skills that learners practice and must do correctly before working with patients. Performance assessments go beyond skills. For example, learners must create, design, produce, integrate, critique, and evaluate. A holistic approach to performance assessment includes a foundation of general and specific knowledge, skills, and values.

Lenburg's (1999) Competency Outcomes and Performance Assessment (COPA) model includes essential outcome competencies relevant to nursing and other health professions. They are:

- Assessment and intervention;
- Communication;
- Critical thinking;
- Teaching;
- Human caring relationships;
- Management;
- Leadership;
- Knowledge integration.

These eight core practice concepts are the framework for the COPA model and can be used to develop performance assessments. It is challenging to construct and evaluate performance assessments. There are opportunities to be creative when developing diverse types of performance assessments. The goal is to develop performance assessments that are summative and are matched to the competencies and associated learning statements.

Types of Performance Assessments

There is a variety of ways to assess performance. Some examples are:

■ **Checklists** are commonly used for psychomotor skills such as patient care activities. An evaluator observes learners as they demonstrate or actually carry out skills. A checklist usually has a pass/fail scale. Each step in a performance needs to be assigned a weight and a passing standard. For example, when taking a blood pressure, there are critical steps that must be taken. Two are correctly inflating the cuff and determining the correct reading. Critical steps could be weighted more than noncritical ones. The learner would need to pass all the critical steps and a certain number of noncritical steps to demonstrate competence. Demonstrating competence requires the learner to meet or exceed the passing standard.

It is also possible to use checklists for oral presentations and video recordings. The skills required include evaluating, critiquing, or summarizing content, concepts, theories, or research. Presentation and communication skills can also be assessed. Students would need to meet all the critical elements such as using presentation technology, making themselves understood, and interacting with the audience.

■ **A rating scale** helps assess different aspects of a performance. A three- to five-point scale is commonly used and can make finer distinctions. It is necessary to set the minimum required performance for each element on the scale. The more clearly the scale is specified, the more reliable (Jacobs & Chase, 1992). Using the example of taking a blood pressure, the rating scale could indicate unsatisfactory, marginal, satisfactory, and excellent. Rubrics would define what is meant by each of the scale descriptors. If a student received a marginal score in an area, a rubric would state what was missing. This is helpful for focusing improvement efforts.

■ **Portfolios** are a collection of student work throughout an entire program. They are especially useful at the end of a course or program. Rubrics must be specific to assure competency in the specified areas. Data are collected over periods of time and can demonstrate progress. Portfolios are especially useful for end-of-program outcome assessment, because the items provide samples of the entire program and can also demonstrate student progress throughout a program. For example, selections of student work, relating to critical thinking, knowledge, or management, from the beginning of the program to the end, can show increasing levels of competence in each area.

■ **Simulations** are becoming more available, and are more sophisticated than in the past. Learners can carry out some skills on mannequins and see results that indicate whether they did the procedure correctly. Computer-based simulation presents all types of situations. Learners then must make choices along a decision tree. Each decision leads them in a certain direction. Foundational knowledge serves as the basis for making a decision. For example, signs and symptoms, health history, and lab values are presented. Critical analysis and synthesis of knowledge is required. As each decision is made, learners receive feedback and have the opportunity to choose another action. If there is a positive outcome at the end of a situation, the learner has demonstrated competence. If not, it is possible to see where bad choices were made and there is the opportunity to continue to practice. Simulations can be used for clinical, management, and teaching situations and include all the primary competencies, as well as the three learning domains. For example, there are simulations used in business training environments. Affective responses, related to values and beliefs, are assessed. Leadership skills are also assessed through simulated role playing. The learners make choices and receive feedback to improve competency in the affective domain (Adkins, 2004).

■ **Journals** are used to demonstrate integration of learning. Reflection and self-assessment are essential to judge and critique performance throughout a career. Learners in all situations can use journaling to express their feelings and how they are reaching their goals. Guidelines for journaling can be structured, open-ended, or somewhere in between. Students in formal education programs may focus on what they are learning, how it will change their thinking when interacting with others, and how they will change their current practice. Journaling may be unstructured or have broad guidelines. For example, a person newly diagnosed with diabetes could write about the physical, emotional, and lifestyle impact of the diagnosis. Setting goals to self-manage their care is helpful. Assessing competence can be done by measuring physical outcomes such as blood glucose, weight, and activity. Affective measures can identify mood, self-confidence, and outlook on life.

■ **Essays** are frequently used to demonstrate critical thinking and synthesis. Learners may have case studies or clinical scenarios that require them to share what they would do in a practice setting. Essays can be used to determine organizational skills, writing ability, and critical analysis. This is a common approach used in higher education. Holistic criteria that look at all the elements can determine competency in the paper itself and the thinking processes that went into developing the topic. Additional skills, such as finding and selecting resources, citing them correctly, organizing the information in a logical sequence, and supporting an argument are essential. For example, students have to write on the topic of health care reform and select a position. What type(s) of health care system should we have in the United States? Research to support a position and the logical presentation of ideas are required to demonstrate competence.

■ **Videotapes** record what learners are doing in a given situation. Their performance in the areas of skills, communication, attitudes, and decisions are assessed. This approach is useful because it conveys what the learner actually did. Evaluators and learners see the same actions and can jointly review the tape. Learners can see areas that need improvement and retape. For evaluators, there is a record of learners' performance. Video technology is especially useful in distance education. Learners can be at different sites and the evaluator can actually see what they did for an assignment (Billings & Halstead, 2005). Table 5.4 summarizes the advantages and challenges of each type of assessment.

Table 5.4

SUMMARY OF ADVANTAGES AND CHALLENGES OF SELECTED TYPES OF PERFORMANCE ASSESSMENTS

PERFORMANCE ASSESSMENTS	ADVANTAGES	CHALLENGES
Checklists	Simple to use. Performance either meets standard or does not.	Does not identify specific areas of performance that need attention. Difficult to make improvements because of lack of specific data.
Rating Scales	Can assess both quantitative and qualitative behaviors related to competencies. Convenient format to make judgments. Offers more options than pass/fail.	May not identify all the complex aspects of a situation. Need to combine observation with questions.
Portfolios	Assesses high-level cognitive and affective domains. Integrates learning. Summative. Broad assessment of learner work.	Time-consuming to collect and grade. Not direct observation. Need clarity on what is being assessed; product or process. Determine responsibility for collection.
Simulations	Assesses high-level cognitive, psychomotor, and affective domains. Integrates learning. Summative. Assesses decision making in a representation of reality.	Requires technology and training to use it. Purpose and grading must be clear.
Journals	Assesses high-level cognitive and affective domains. Integrates learning. Summative.	Time-consuming to assess. Students may be frustrated by assignments. Grading rubric may not be clear.
Essays	Assesses high-level cognitive and affective domains. Integrates learning. Summative.	Limited assessment of content. Time-consuming to grade. Reliability of assessment may be difficult.
Videotapes	Assesses high-level cognitive and affective domains. Integrates learning. Summative. Assesses actual learner performance. Good for distance-learning programs.	Requires technology and training to use it. Reliability of assessment may be difficult.

Adapted from Billings and Halstead (2005).

Table 5.5

EXAMPLES OF PRIMARY AND SECONDARY COMPETENCIES AND LEARNING STATEMENTS

CORE PRIMARY PRACTICE COMPETENCIES	SECONDARY COMPETENCIES	LEARNING STATEMENTS
Critical thinking	Ethical reasoning: The learner will have a broad knowledge of ethical principles.	Determine an appropriate ethical principle for the selected nursing practice dilemma. Apply the selected ethical principle to the selected nursing practice dilemma. Evaluate the outcomes of the application of the ethical principle to the selected nursing practice dilemma.

Steps in Developing Performance Assessments

Step 1

The first step in developing performance assessments is to organize the competencies and the specific learning statements. In this example, the COPA model describes the eight core primary practice competencies. From the primary competencies, secondary competencies are developed. Under each secondary competency are learning statements. For each secondary competency, there may be two-to-four learning statements.

Table 5.5 provides examples of primary and secondary competencies and learning statements.

Because there is a focus on preparing nursing and other health professional graduates for the real world of practice, groups are convened to develop the competencies and the related learning statements. Group members are often working in practice settings, are leaders in health care organizations, or educators with expertise in specific content areas. Additionally, professional and regulatory standards and best practices, based on evidence, are used in the development processes.

The processes are the same for creating performance assessments for patient/client education and staff-development programs. Multiple sources of information are used to develop competencies and learning statements that reflect concepts in the COPA model. The expected competencies for these groups are: assessment and intervention, communication, critical thinking, management, and knowledge integration.

The use of diverse individuals and resources is different from a group of faculty or an individual using one source to develop test items. Having wide participation assures the competencies are aligned to clinical practice, are current, and are evidence-based.

In order to assure the development processes are uniform, the participants are trained by the professional staff in the organization. The staff is well versed in the processes and experts in test development and psychometric principles. A common language and format is used. The goal is to have consistency and uniformity (Nicastro & Moreton, 2008).

Step 2

An essential part of developing performance assessments is determining the format, information and directions to be included, and rubrics. Learners need consistent approaches to performance assessments. Each time they work on an assessment, they can expect the elements will be the same. They do not need to figure out how to approach the assessment or spend time and effort understanding how it will be graded.

Step 3

The specific elements of the performance-assessment task are finalized. There is a coding system to organize the competencies in their primary and secondary groups with the associated learning statements. Common elements listed are:

■ The primary competency;
■ The secondary competency;
■ The associated learning statements;

■ Background information to provide a context for the assessment (e.g., to assess ethical reasoning, a scenario or case is provided. The goal is to use foundational knowledge to resolve the ethical dilemma presented);

■ Include a suggested length for the paper or project. Example: Complete a six-to-eight-page paper that includes all the areas listed in the assessment;

■ Resources are identified for the learner. These may include readings, multimedia, and course materials. Examples: review ethical theories, review ethical principles, and review APA style for the paper and reference list;

■ The performance assignment or project is described in detail. Learners are given step-by-step directions to complete the assignment. Examples:

1. Choose one ethical theory and provide a rationale for its selection;
2. Cite two sources to support your choice of ethical theory;
3. Choose two ethical principles and provide a rationale related to the theory;
4. Analyze how the principles provide a framework for resolving the ethical dilemma;
5. Determine the key persons and their roles involved in resolving the dilemma;
6. Compare two potential outcomes and relate them to the principles;
7. Cite two sources to support the selected outcomes;
8. Predict the impact of the outcomes on resolving the dilemma;
9. Evaluate one outcome to determine how it matches the theory and principles selected (Burkhardt and Nathaniel, 2002).
10. Confirm grammar, punctuation, and sentence structure is correct;
11. Confirm APA format is used for citations in the text and the reference list.

■ Notes can also be added under a section to clarify what is meant or give further instructions. Example: Choose two ethical principles and provide a rationale.
Note: You need to determine which ethical principles best support the resolution of an ethical dilemma related to making health care decisions;

- A list of references and Websites can be added;
- Attachments such as rubrics, forms to complete, and any other items students need to complete an assignment.

Step 4

It is essential that performance tasks have specific, clear rubrics for each of the areas in the assessment. The persons who develop the assessments also complete the rubrics. There are several deliberations related to rubric development:

- A common scoring framework is developed for all the rubrics. This means there is the same number of categories and the same terms used. Example: A 4-point scale with the same terms to describe them: 1 = poor, 2 = fair, 3 = average, and 4 = above average.
- A passing standard (requirement) is identified. Example: A student's paper or project must be receive a 3 (average) on all the areas of the assignment OR receive an average of 3 on the assignment.
- Options for students who fall below the passing standard should be explained. Example: A student who earns an overall score of 2 will have the option of making one revision to each of the areas with scores of 1 and 2.
- The language used to define the expectations for each area must be clear. Example:

1. Choose two ethical principles and provide a rationale that relates to the theory:

1 = poor. The learner only selects one ethical principle and does not state a rationale;

2 = fair. The learner selects two ethical principles and provides illogical rationales;

3 = average. The learner selects two ethical principles and provides rationales to support the selections;.

4 = above average. The learner selects two ethical principles and provides rationales to support the selection and relates them to the dilemma.

Students receive the rubrics to prepare for the assessment. They know what is expected in the completed assignment. The graders/ evaluators also have the rubrics. In addition, they also have grader/ evaluator notes. O'Brien, Franks, and Stowe (2008) provide an example of a rubric-based method to assess pharmacy students' case presentations.

Step 5

Another critical part of the performance-assessment process is grading. It involves both the persons who grade the assessments and the processes used:

■ Objectivity in grading is always a concern of students and faculty. The strategy used for performance assessments is to have the persons who develop the assessments also develop the grader notes. The subject experts develop the grader notes along with the assessments and rubrics. They are the persons who have the expertise. This process also supports coherency among all the parts. There is not any contact between the developers and graders.

■ Grader notes provide the graders/evaluators with information and examples so they have an understanding of the topic and types of responses. They are able to consistently grade multiple assessments that cover the same topic. Example: Choose two ethical principles and provide a rationale that relates to the theory.

Grader Notes. Grader notes provide direction for the evaluators to determine the range of responses that are acceptable. Two examples are:

■ The scenario for this assessment addresses an issue of who should make decisions about patient/client care. The principle of autonomy supports guidelines for patient and family decision making. This includes informed consent, avoiding staff paternalism, and dealing with patient/client noncompliance issues (Burkhardt & Nathaniel, 2002).

■ Another principle that supports decision making is beneficence. This principle requires health care providers to act in ways that benefit patients/clients. Such acts are morally and legally required. This principle requires nurses to actually do good, do no harm, and advocate for patients/clients (Burkhardt & Nathaniel, 2002).

Graders/evaluators are trained by the professional staff. They may come to a site or have online sessions. They have backgrounds as educators and are experts in a variety of subject areas. The graders/ evaluators may work from home and have regular communication with the professional staff.

In formal academic settings, learners work with their assigned faculty mentors to determine when they are ready for an assessment. The faculty mentor schedules the assessments. Learners may submit the completed assessments electronically. They receive feedback and review the results with their mentor. There is an appeal process if they think the grade should be different.

In nonacademic settings, such as patient education and staff development classes, the assessment processes may be different. Learners may take home their assignments, complete them in the class, or go online to complete them.

There are many options for computerized educational programs that include assessments, so learners receive immediate feedback. The learners can also review their answers and retake the assessment.

Step 6

Evaluation of performance assessments includes determining validity and reliability. As described earlier in the chapter, there are different types of validity and reliability. Validity is established early in the performance-assessment development process. The inclusion of panels of experts from education, practice, and testing and measurement assures there is content and criterion validity. Construct validity is supported by tying assessment outcomes to competencies.

Reliability estimates the consistency of a measure; does the instrument measure the same way each time it is used? Roberts, Newble, Jolly, Reed, and Hampton (2006) discussed issues in standardizing clinical and other types of competency assessments. Establishing reliability requires the identification and reduction of measurement errors and biases. One problem is that content is not specific, and therefore, it is difficult to assess what is desired. Testing samples of assessments for long periods of time and having multiple measures increases reliability.

Another approach to establishing reliability is to use Cronbach's alpha statistical test to measure the internal consistency of an assessment. A result of 0.8 or higher is positive. Different parts of an assessment, such as individual assessment areas and results from individual evaluators, can also be determined. Interrater reliability can be established between evaluators using Pearson correlations. Stability, equivalence, and internal consistency measures all provide data to help ensure assessments are more reliable.

Validity and reliability data can be collected and analyzed in different ways. It is critical to establish program or course processes that are used consistently. Examples include:

■ An assessment review group that meets annually to review previous data, share changes in standards, regulations, guidelines, and best practices. Assessments are revised, based on the data and new information.

■ Standardized performance assessments, comparable with program/course competency assessments, are administered. The results from individual students and aggregated data are compared.

■ Qualitative approaches, such as observation and interviews, can be structured to determine whether the results are credible, dependable, and can be confirmed. The qualitative data can be matched to quantitative data to determine whether individuals and groups have achieved the primary and secondary competencies (Trochim, 2005).

■ The reliability of performance assessment grading can be established by comparing the results from different evaluators (Trochim, 2005);

■ Simulations to assess competency are becoming more widely used. Medical education has been a leader. Simulations provide the opportunity to assess what learners would actually do, rather than assessing what they know, or how they would do. One reason for using simulations is their high degree of reliability. The evaluation problems are presented in the same manner, time after time. The ability to reproduce the same situation is especially important in high-stakes decisions (e.g., certification and licensure) (Scalese, Obeso, & Issenberg, 2008).

For all the processes described in this chapter, each organization has review and approval procedures in place. The goal is to make certain

Exhibit 5.1

Core Primary Practice Competencies (select 1 from the COPA Model):

_____

Secondary Competencies (develop one related to the core primary competency):

Learning Statements (develop one for an objective assessment and one for a performance assessment)

Objective	Performance
1. Objective Assessment	
2. Performance Assessment	

the assessments are complete and meet quality standards for content, measurement principles, readability, clarity, and form. Continuous improvement processes are essential to maintaining the quality of the assessments used to verify competency.

SUMMARY

Assessment development is an important step in the competency-based learning process. When assessment items directly measure performance of identified competencies, learners know what the expected performance level is and have the opportunity to demonstrate the appropriate behaviors. Two popular methods for setting standard cut scores are Angoff and Bookmark. Groups of experts use their judgment to determine the minimum acceptable score. Angoff is used frequently with multiple-choice items, whereas Bookmark can be used with both multiple-choice and open-response items. Assuring assessments are valid and reliable increases confidence in assessment results.

CHAPTER 5 ACTIVITY

The previous chapters have presented the information and processes you needed to start planning and developing a competency-based education or course. Chapter 5 provides specific guidelines for selecting assessments. Review your responses to the chapter 3 questions. Use the competency and learning statements you developed in chapter 4 to determine the related assessments.

Use Exhibit 5.1 to develop a primary practice competency, a secondary competency, two learning statements, one objective assessment, and one performance assessment.

REFERENCES

Adkins, S. (2004, February). Beneath the tip of the iceberg. (cover story). *Training + Development, 58*(2), 28–33. Retrieved May 2, 2009, from http://goliath.ecnext.com/coms2/gi_0199-524274/Beneath-the-tip-of-the.html

Burkhardt, M. A., & Nathaniel, A. K. (2002). *Ethics & issues in contemporary nursing.* Clifton Park, NJ: Delmar Thompson Learning.

Billings, D. M., & Halstead, J. A. (2005). *Teaching in nursing: A guide for faculty.* St. Louis, MO: Elsevier Saunders.

Forehand, M. (2008). *Bloom's taxonomy.* Retrieved August 8, 2009, from http://projects. coe.uga.edu/epltt/index.php?title=Bloom%27s_Taxonomy

Giraud, G., Impara, J., & Plake, B. (2005, July). Teachers' conceptions of the target examinee in Angoff standard setting. *Applied Measurement in Education, 18*(3), 223–232.

Hill, H., Dean, C., & Goffney, I. (2007). Focus article: Assessing elemental and structural validity: Data from teachers, non-teachers, and mathematicians. *Measurement, 5*(23), 81–92.

Jacobs, L. C., & Chase, C. I. (1992). *Developing and using tests effectively.* San Francisco: Jossey-Bass

Johnson, R. R., Squires, J. R., & Whitney, D. (2002). Setting the standard for passing professional certification examinations. Retrieved May 2, 2009, from http://209.85.173.132/search?q=cache:XwcE-9X39nsJ:www.fma.org/FMAOnline/certifications.pdf+Setting+the+stan dard+for+passing+professional+Certification+examinations.&cd=1&hl=en&ct=clnk&gl=us&client=firefox-a

Lenburg, C. B. (1999). Redesigning expectations for initial and continuing competence for contemporary practice. *Online Journal of Issues in Nursing. 4*(3). Retrieved Febru-

ary 18, 2009, from
http://www.nursingworld.org/MainMenuCategories/ANAMarketplace/
ANAPeriodicals/OJIN/TableofContents/Volume41999/No2Sep1999/Redesi
gningExpectationsforInitialandContinuingCompetence.aspx

Lin, J. (n.d.). *The Bookmark standard setting procedure: Strengths and weaknesses.* Alberta, Canada: The Centre for Research in Applied Measurement and Evaluation. Retrieved August 8, 2009, from http://www.education.ualberta.ca/educ/psych/crame/files/standard_setting.pdf

Nicastro, G., & Moreton, K. M. (2008). Development of quality performance tasks at Western Governors University. *Assessment Update, 20*(1), 8–9.

O'Brien, C. E., Franks, A. M., & Stowe, C. D. (2008). Multiple rubric-based assessments of student case presentations. *American Journal of Pharmaceutical Education, 72*(3), 1–7.

Roberts, C., Newble, D., Jolly, B., Reed, M., & Hampton, K. (2006). Assuring the quality of high-stakes undergraduate assessments of clinical competence. *Medical Teacher, 28*(6), 535–543.

Scalese, R. J., Obeso, V. T., & Issenberg, S. B. (2008). Simulation technology for skills training and competency assessment in medical education. *Journal of General Internal Medicine, 23*(1), 46–49.

Schagen, I., & Bragshaw, J. (2003, September). *Modelling item difficulty for Bookmark standard setting.* Paper presented at the British Educational Research Association Annual Conference, Heriot-Watt University, Edinburgh, Scotland, UK.

Snelgrove, S., & Slater, J. (2003, September). Approaches to learning: psychometric testing of a study process questionnaire. *Journal of Advanced Nursing, 43*(5), 496–505.

Trochim, W. M. K. (2005). *Research methods: The concise knowledge base.* Cincinnati, OH: Atomic Dog Publishing.

Verheggen, M., Muijtiens, A., & Van Os, J. (2008). Is an Angoff standard an indication of minimal competence of examinees or of judges? *Advanced Health Science Education Theory Practice, 13*(2), 203–211.

Voorhees, R. A. (Ed.). (2001). *Measuring what matters: Competency-based learning models in higher education.* San Francisco: Jossey-Bass.

ADDITIONAL RESOURCES

Assessment Terminology: A Glossary of Useful Terms
http://www.newhorizons.org/strategies/assess/terminology.htm
Competency-Based Training (CBT): In a CBT system, the unit of progression is mastery of specific knowledge and skills and is learner- or participant-centered. *http://www.reproline.jhu.edu/english/6read/6training/cbt/cbt.htm*
A Power Point® slide presentation: Determining the value of simulation training within nurse education: A literature review. From the Bristol Medical Simulation Centre. Contact details: *sarah.@bmsc.co.uk* Visit *www.bmsc.co.uk*

Toolbox of Assessment Methods (describes different methods) *http://www.acgme.org/
   Outcome/assess/Toolbox.pdf*
Western Governors University (WGU) is a leader in competency-based education. The
   January/February 2008, issue of *Assessment Update* is devoted to the processes
   used to develop all the programs.

6

Data Collection and Use to Verify Achievement of Outcomes

MARION G. ANEMA

OVERVIEW

This chapter moves from the development of objective and performance assessments for individual learners to a focus on program or course outcome assessment. It is vital for learners and teachers to have evidence of each learner's achievement. Another essential piece is to review the entire course or program. Improvements cannot be made by reviewing individual results. Combining or aggregating individual outcome data provides the big picture of what is happening in a course or program.

The stakeholders have been previously identified. They provide support and leadership for the programs and need to know whether the outcomes have been achieved. Each course, program, and organization develops criteria for outcomes. The outcomes provide details of what was accomplished and relates them to mission, regulations, and standards.

Processes for establishing outcome assessments and selecting data are described in this chapter. The importance of using the data for improvement, and strategies for doing so, are discussed. Finally, approaches to organizing and sharing the data are covered.

INTRODUCTION

The concept of assessing the outcomes of courses, programs, agencies, organizations, and institutions is fairly new. Program outcome assessment is built on the assessment of elements within a program. When an educational offering is first developed, external and internal factors are considered. When a program is implemented, it is hoped that the expected outcomes will be achieved. The goal of program outcome assessment is to determine whether the program met those expectations.

Ideally, the program outcome-assessment plan is constructed during program development. For example, a diabetic education program may set goals (benchmarks) to begin with a specified number of participants, have 80% of the participants complete the program, and after one year, 60% of the participants maintain appropriate blood glucose, weight, blood pressure, and exercise levels. The actual outcomes of the program are compared with the expected outcomes. The information identifies both the positive outcomes and the areas for improvement. The aim is to achieve the benchmarks in all the different areas and make sure current standards are met.

PURPOSES OF OUTCOME EVALUATION

Common purposes of outcome evaluation are to:

- Review the entire educational offering to determine how the pieces fit together.
  Example: A diabetic education program has six modules. They were developed for learners to progress on a continuum of knowledge about their condition to self-management. Within each module, the content moves from simple to complex. A review could include looking at responses from the participants about the organization of the program. Knowledgeable nurses or student nurses could also complete the modules and use rubrics to provide input.
- Examine how the course/program outcomes support the mission, goals, and desired organizational outcomes.

Example: Compare the organizational information with the program outcomes. If the organization has a mission to meet the needs of diverse groups, then the participants should have those characteristics. If the program was presented only in English and the diverse groups in the community have different languages, then changes and improvements are needed. Additional stakeholders may need to be added to the program-planning process.

■ Analyze whether the educational offering was implemented as planned.

Example: The organization uses computer technology in all areas of its operations. The diabetic education program was developed from this perspective. During implementation, it became apparent that participants needed extensive training and some became discouraged and dropped out. It was apparent to the staff that changes were needed in this area. Other low-tech options should be developed and used.

■ Assess whether the different types of resources were used efficiently.

Example: Every organization is concerned about how their resources are used. Attendance records could show the number of participants at each session, multiple sessions could be collapsed or new sections added. The number of staff at each session could be compared with the number of participants. The days, times, and locations of the education program can also be reviewed to determine whether the resources were congruent with the needs.

■ Interpret outcome data to determine strengths and improvements needed.

Example: Look at all the data and compare them with the different benchmarks. Also, summarize the positive outcomes and prioritize the areas needing improvement. Determine whether any new initiatives are needed. A concise presentation of the outcomes provides a holistic, readable document. Stakeholders and decision makers know what happened. Sharing the information in the media brings positive attention to the organization, increases interest, and possibly brings opportunities for additional support.

■ Justify decisions made to improve the educational offering (Billings & Halstead, 2005).

Example: The outcomes of the diabetic education program indicated that there was not enough space for all the people who wanted to attend. The participants who completed the program wanted to continue with a support group so they could maintain their individual outcomes. The argument could be made that people who control their diabetes have fewer complications and associated costs than those who do not manage their condition. From the program outcomes, develop a plan to make improvements. Use the same steps presented in earlier chapters to gain support and specifically identify the new resources needed.

The purposes can be applied to any type of educational program. Outcome-assessment data support celebrations of achievements, directions for improvements, and guidance for new initiatives. In academic nursing programs, there is always a concern about the National Council Licensure Examination-Registered Nurse (NCLEX-RN) pass rate. Rather than rely on anecdotal comments and conjecture, data from several sources can provide a focus for changes to improve the pass rate. Staff development is very costly. If nurses and other providers are not competent to practice after completing programs, they may complain, make mistakes, or resign. Systematic methods to collect, analyze, and use data for continuous improvement is required.

EXTERNAL AND INTERNAL REQUIREMENTS FOR PROGRAM OUTCOME ASSESSMENT

Today, there are many standards, regulations, and professional groups that provide frameworks for evaluation and accreditation. Every educational institution and health care provider in the United States and throughout the world has to meet licensing, certification, approval, and regulatory guidelines to be able to provide their services. The individuals providing services and practicing in these environments also need to meet specific guidelines. It would be impossible to list all the different entities because there are so many. The following are examples of different types of organizations that have guidelines or requirements that influence what is included in program outcome-assessment plans. The information is from their Websites, which are listed at the end of the chapter.

■ **The Joint Commission.** The mission of The Joint Commission is to continuously improve the safety and quality of care provided to the public through the provision of health care accreditation and related services that support performance improvement in health care organizations. Their services include accreditation, certification, standards, patient safety guidelines, performance measures, and public policy reports.

The Joint Commission also provides health care staffing services certification that provides a comprehensive evaluation of key processes, such as verifying the credentials and competencies of health care staff;

■ **The Commission on Collegiate Nursing Education (CCNE).** The CCNE is an autonomous accrediting agency contributing to the improvement of the public's health. CCNE ensures the quality and integrity of baccalaureate and graduate education programs preparing effective nurses;

■ **The National Commission for Health Education Credentialing, Inc. (NCHEC).** The NCHEC's mission is to improve the practice of health education and to serve the public and profession of health education by certifying health education specialists, promoting professional development, and strengthening professional preparation and practice.

   ○ NCHEC develops and administers a national competency-based examination, develops standards for professional preparation, and provides continuing education programs;

■ **The National Certification Board for Diabetes Educators (NCBDE).** The NCBDE's mission is to develop, maintain, and protect the certification process and the CDE Certified Diabetes Educator® credential. The NCBDE recognizes and advances the specialty practice of diabetes education. The CDE credential demonstrates that the certified health care professional possesses distinct and specialized knowledge, thereby promoting quality care for persons with diabetes;

■ **The National League for Nursing Academic Nurse Educator Certification Program (CNE).** The CNE recognizes excellence in the advanced specialty role of the academic nurse educator. The goals of CNE certification are to recognize academic nursing education as a specialty area of practice, recognize specialized knowledge, skills, abilities, and excellence in practice, strengthen the use of core competencies, and contribute to professional development;

■ **Physical Therapy Licensing** is approved by the American Physical Therapy Association's Commission on Accreditation in Physical Therapy Education. All physical therapists must pass the National Physical Therapist Examination (NPTE) developed by the Federation of State Boards of Physical Therapy. Each state may have additional requirements for licensure.

Each organization, institution, and discipline has its own specialized standards and guidelines that dictate outcomes. It is the responsibility of program developers to determine the best ways to assess the outcomes. In the end, there has to be a coherent outcome-assessment plan that fully communicates the program goals, determines to what extent the goals were reached, and decides what improvements will be made. There are different theories, models, and approaches to putting together an outcome-assessment plan.

THEORIES AND MODELS FOR PROGRAM EVALUATION

There are two approaches commonly used to organize program evaluation plans. A theory-based approach focuses on one or more theories that provide a framework for program evaluation.

Example: A diabetic education program could be developed using normative goal (outcome) evaluation theory. The question is what do the stakeholders want to accomplish? Stakeholders can participate in the process through focus groups, surveys, and other techniques, such as the Delphi process. The Delphi process consists of several rounds of sharing ideas. The process can start with the main question. The stakeholders submit their ideas during the first round. A small group organizes the information and sends another round with the ideas ranked. The process continues with more rounds until there is consensus about what they want to accomplish. The desired goals and outcomes are determined. Stakeholders must reach consensus. Next, the consistency between goals and program activities is examined. During the development of program activities, their consistency with the goals is compared. The outcomes can also be compared with organizational elements. This theoretical approach can be used during program development, and also for a program that was previously developed and needs to have the outcomes assessed (Billings & Halstead, 2005).

A second approach is method oriented, rather than theory oriented. A method-based approach primarily emphasizes the collection of quantitative data. This approach is useful in courses or programs where limited information is needed (Billings & Halstead, 2005).

Example: A surgical center opened 1 year ago. It is part of a larger system that has comprehensive assessment processes in place. The goal is to determine patient satisfaction with the services. This is a limited assessment. The nursing director selects patient satisfaction items from existing ones and adds any new ones needed. A paper survey is mailed and others are sent by e-mail. An additional assessment method would be to make phone calls to randomly selected patients. That process would collect qualitative data. The outcome data from the surgical center becomes part of the overall system-assessment process, with comparisons and benchmarks to other units.

The theory-focused model is widely used, especially in academic educational programs. The institution or program can select a theory or blend theories that fit with their mission, goals, and discipline values and beliefs. A theory-driven model also can be comprehensive, to assess all elements of an educational program. The next section presents the elements of a theory-driven approach to an academic nursing program outcome assessment.

ELEMENTS OF COMPREHENSIVE PROGRAM OUTCOME ASSESSMENTS

A comprehensive academic program outcome assessment is usually theory-based, because one or more theories support all the different required evaluation instrument elements. A plan is developed to organize and track all the evaluation activities. Program background information is presented first.

Program Background Information: The program example is a bachelor of science of nursing (BSN) program. The public, comprehensive university has about 10,000 students. The majority of programs are at the undergraduate level, with a few master's level programs in teacher education and business. The nursing program has 1,200 students. Six hundred of them are in prenursing courses, and the others are taking nursing courses. The nursing program has two years of general education requirements and two years of nursing courses. The university has an outcome-assessment plan. The nursing faculty will use information from that plan and add nursing-specific requirements.

It is useful to organize a plan around accreditation standards, because all the elements for outcome assessment are included in the standards. Accreditation evaluators find it helpful to have the diverse elements organized accordingly. The faculty is updating their current plan to prepare for nursing reaccreditation in 4 years. They are using the CCNE standards. The parts of an evaluation plan are described. A sample of elements and format for this type of evaluation plan is presented in Table 6.1. The table includes only a small part of a comprehensive plan. A complete plan would have several standards and the key elements or competencies, with multiple assessments for each. The first two-to-three pages would be an introduction to the plan, how it was developed, and the format. A plan like this could be 30–40 pages long, depending on the complexity of the evaluation plan, the number of standards, and the number of assessments used for each area.

Evaluation Framework

Example: For the BSN program, different types of a theory-driven model are selected. Table 6.2 presents how Chen's theory-driven evaluation types are suitable for selected components of the evaluation plan (Billings & Halstead, 2005). Each program which uses a theory-driven model needs to select the types of evaluation that fit with the components being evaluated.

Assignment of Responsibilities

A program-evaluation plan is a major undertaking for any organization or institution. Although there should be broad participation in evaluation, there needs to be a structure for developing and implementing an evaluation plan. Initially, there should be broad participation to discuss ideas and make the major decisions. A core group of people should be assigned overall responsibility for the project. The core group can individually take on specific tasks and also lead others. They can delegate various aspects and closely monitor what is happening. It is essential to include persons with different types of expertise. Experts can have different levels of participation, depending on the phase of

Table 6.1

SAMPLE OUTCOME-ASSESSMENT PLAN

Standard IV–Program Effectiveness: Student Performance and Faculty Accomplishments

Definition: The program is fulfilling its mission, philosophy, and expected outcomes congruent with expected student outcomes.

Outcomes: Student performance accomplishments are summarized in program documents and reports.

The program is effective in fulfilling its mission, goals, and expected outcomes. Actual student learning outcomes are consistent with the mission, goals, and expected outcomes of the program.

Key Elements:	Document or indicator evidence	Responsible person, delegated to	Frequency	Assessment method	Assessment of method (reliability, validity, specificity)	Submission of report	Actions based on assessment data (development, maintenance, revision)
Standard IV program effectiveness, student performance, and faculty accomplishments							
Student outcome data include NCLEX-RN pass rates, standardized exam rates, and employer satisfaction	Standardized CH exam	CH faculty team leader	End of course	Individual exam scores are aggregated	Exam is specifically developed for students completing a CH course. Reliability and validity have been established with national norms by the testing service.	Faculty, school curriculum committee, BSN program director, dean	The current assessment was maintained because data showed continued improvement from three years ago to the present.

Table 6.2

THEORY-DRIVEN EVALUATION TYPES COMPARED WITH SELECTED COMPONENTS OF THE EVALUATION PLAN

EVALUATION TYPES	SELECTED COMPONENTS
Normative outcome evaluation (goal evaluation)	Mission and goal evaluation
Normative treatment evaluation (was program implemented as planned?)	Curriculum and teaching effectiveness evaluation
Implementation environment evaluation (how was the program delivered?)	Learner dimension Participant dimension
Participant Dimension (evaluates participant characteristics, demographics, and response to the program.)	
Impact evaluation (did the program achieve goals; desired and unintended outcomes are examined?)	Outcomes assessment

Adapted from Billings and Halstead (2005).

evaluation. These people can have different levels of participation during different phases.

Example: One approach that faculty and staff feel is fair is to have the work spread out. Although there is broad participation at all levels, there needs to be someone in charge and responsible for the plan. A faculty person may have released time to do this. If there are several administrators or directors, the responsibilities for all types of assessment may be part of their job. In a program where there is one course offered, the person responsible for the program could manage the outcome-assessment processes. It is also very helpful to have an administrative or staff person providing support and tracking what is done and what still needs to be done.

Example: In the BSN program, the choice was made to give a faculty member released time. This choice fits with the program because it has a very flat organizational structure. The dean has overall responsibility for the program. Experienced course and level faculty head up teams.

Professor Jones is an experienced faculty member, has provided leadership for previous reporting activities, and works well with nursing faculty and other departments. An administration assistant, Ms. Janet Moore, is assigned half time to support the outcome-assessment activities.

Time Frame for Evaluation Processes

The time frame for completing a total evaluation project is often determined by external evaluators, such as accrediting and regulatory agencies. In those situations, a timeline is developed, working backwards. Events like a site visit, submission of a self-study, and deadlines for submitting reports determine what needs to be done, and by what time.

If the total evaluation is on a smaller scale, then less time and fewer resources are needed. Reasons for doing smaller scale evaluations are reviewing a new program, reevaluating selected outcomes to determine changes from the previous assessments, or doing a review after standards or guidelines were changed. If a comprehensive plan is organized according to standards or methods, it is possible to select the elements needed because the bases are developed. It is always possible that standards and guidelines may change during the project. That may require making new decisions, adding evaluation processes, and expanding into new areas. A time frame may be as short as six months or as long as two-to-three years. Within the program evaluation plan are specific assessment pieces, such as end of course or program evaluations, annual performance evaluations, and follow up at set times. All these pieces fit together into the comprehensive plan.

Example: The BSN faculty know there have been changes in the accreditation standards since the last cycle. They also know they need three years of outcome data and they must submit the self-study about six months before the site visit. The time frame is adequate, but planning to get all the tasks done before it is time to submit the self-study will help them. During the first year, they will set up their structure for managing the data collection and related processes. Templates for different parts of the self-study can begin to be filled in, such as the university mission and philosophy. It is easier to have a good draft updated as new data are available, rather than start from the beginning several months before the self-study needs to be ready.

Each program which uses a theory-driven model needs to select the types of evaluations that fit with the components being reviewed. A major decision in deciding the next component of an evaluation plan is evaluation methods.

Evaluation Methods

Total program evaluation requires multiple methods to assess all the different program components. There are many options, and it may be difficult to decide on methods. Organizations may also believe that the more sophisticated and complicated the assessment methods, the more impressive they are, and may be trying to measure elements that are not important. Determine the essential areas of assessment.

Accreditation and regulatory standards and guidelines provide a focus. Tables and charts can be developed to make comparisons. Use university assessments forms and adapt or add parts that are discipline specific. Unless the program is new, assessment methods should be in place.

Qualitative methods are appropriate when the value of programs or experiences is desired. For example, clinical experiences are often pass/fail. Quantitative data include number of times a student had clinical experiences, the types of patients, and procedures. Qualitative data can also be collected to determine whether the experiences increased their self-confidence, developed congenial relations with staff, and had positive responses from the patient for the care they received. Selected examples of assessment methods are provided in Table 6.3.

Example: The BSN faculty selected the methods listed in Table 6.3, because there is a good fit between the methods and the components. Faculty also wanted to collect both quantitative and qualitative data. They believed it would broaden the perspectives on experiences and activities that are part of the program. Student program satisfaction is assessed using an instrument with a scale. They have to select from four choices: strongly disagree, disagree, agree, strongly agree. A qualitative method expands what students can share by responding to open-ended questions and giving examples.

The data have been collected electronically so results can be analyzed quickly. For example, student, faculty, employer, and alumni surveys were all submitted electronically. The results from individuals are kept confidential by the computer center staff.

Table 6.3

PROGRAM ELEMENTS AND SAMPLE ASSESSMENT METHODS

PROGRAM ELEMENTS	ASSESSMENT METHODS
Mission and goals	Compare themes from organization and program missions and goals. Compare accreditation standards with program mission and goals.
Curriculum	Compare curriculum elements with current accreditation standards. Review specific outcomes to curriculum elements, such as course grades to standardized test results.
Course	Compare individual course outcomes with program benchmarks related to retention and NCLEX-RN pass rates. Diabetic course outcomes related to changes in behavior and benchmark values for weight, blood glucose, BP, and activity.
Teaching effectiveness	University and program teaching effectiveness assessment form, compare nursing faculty outcomes with university faculty outcomes. Nursing-specific forms for peer and student input.
Learning resources	Compare nursing resources with resources for similar programs and external standards for learning resources, such as library holdings and services.
Student learning	Course assessments, standardized exams, and end-of-program exit exams, portfolios, reflection journals, written assignments, care plans, clinical evaluations, self-evaluations, and presentations.
Faculty	Compare university expectations for teaching, scholarship, and service. Examine faculty curriculum vita (CV) and faculty university outcomes form for each of the areas.
Employer	Surveys to identify strengths/weaknesses and satisfaction with graduates.
Alumni	Surveys to identify strengths/weaknesses and satisfaction with program six months after graduation and periodically thereafter.

Adapted from Billings and Halstead, 2005.

Methods to Analyze Data

The majority of data will be descriptive. It will describe the sample from which data were collected. For example, faculty outcomes related to teaching scholarship and service can be organized and summarized as percentages. If 40% of the BSN program faculty participated in service, how does this segment rank compared with the total university faculty? What is the benchmark or goal set for all faculty? If the university goal is 80% participation, then nursing faculty needs to increase their activities in this area.

Example: The BSN program requires that students have an average of 75% to pass a course. The *mean* is the average of a group of scores. It is useful to know how a group scored overall. The mean is affected by extreme scores, very high or low. If most students have average scores of 90%, that may indicate the exams are too easy. If the average scores on an exam are below 60%, it may indicate the exam was too difficult or the content was not presented and discussed. The *median* is the point at which half the scores are below it and half are above. An advantage of this measure is that very high or low scores do not affect it. Collecting qualitative data is another approach.

QUALITATIVE DATA

Focus groups are one way to collect qualitative data. An interviewer can have a set of structured questions for the group members who had the same experiences. Individual student conferences and journaling during the program can also address reflections of experiences. The data can be analyzed using:

■ A template analysis that is highly structured to provide a systematic and standardized approach. An advantage is it is simple to use, is efficient, and it is easily taught to faculty;

■ An editing analysis that has the evaluator focus on meaningful segments to discover relationships and interactions. This approach requires more training;

■ The least structured approach is immersion analysis, when the evaluator becomes completely immersed. Experience and intuition are required (Houser, 2008).

Example: The end-of-semester assessments are done, and faculty are particularly interested in comparing the qualitative data and matching quantitative data related to the first nursing course. They want more information about why the attrition has dropped in that course. The faculty believe they can use the editing analysis approach if they have some training. Two faculty members have experience with qualitative analysis and will also check results.

When evaluating a program, individual learner outcomes are not the focus. The goal is to describe how all the different elements are implemented. The process of aggregating the data places the focus on the broader theme rather than on specific outcomes. It is also important to link the different elements of the program together.

Example: The university and the nursing program are on a mission to have a diverse student body. Nursing faculty serve on a university-wide committee to review marketing/recruitment materials and activities. They find that:

- Materials illustrate different ethnic and cultural groups;
- Events are held at a variety of sites to attract diverse students;
- Outcomes data show a steady increase in student diversity, but the numbers are not reflective of the population in the community and surrounding areas;
- Student support services are in place;
- The nursing curriculum addresses diversity in the populations served;
- Students are excused from class to observe religious holidays;
- Faculty throughout the university and in nursing represent different cultural and ethnic groups;
- The committee suggested that a student mentor system be implemented to have prospective students spend a day on campus, and have contact with a mentor student by email. This proposal is being considered by administration.

Data from all these different sources provide a comprehensive view and establishes coherence within the program. The next step is to put data in formats that are useful.

DISPLAYING DATA

An essential part of a program-evaluation plan is to share the data in ways others can understand it; this includes summaries of numeric values, compares summaries with other outcomes, and presents graphics as appropriate. Tables and charts are efficient ways to present a large amount of data in a small space. Data are displayed so they are easy to read. Comparison of data is also a benefit of tables and charts (American Psychological Association, 2001).

Program evaluation is usually done annually; for instance, at the end of an academic year. Additionally, data should be compared for at least three years.

Example: Professor Jones is responsible for developing the plan and works with Ms. Moore. They discuss ways to present the data. They look at the last university self-study and the previous one for nursing. They first select the nursing outcome data that are a subset of university outcomes, and includes retention, graduation, and class ranks. They develop tables to compare the nursing results with the university to determine whether they are meeting the benchmarks in these areas. The dean will review the information and forward it to university administrators. Professor Jones will continue this process and make comparisons of other data with national and state outcomes. The data for the year will be entered in the faculty notes, reviewed, and added to the comprehensive evaluation plan. Once the data are organized and displayed, there can be discussion about trends from year to year.

TRENDING

Looking at the aggregated data each year and comparing at least three years' worth of data is part of a continuous improvement process. Outcomes are reviewed each year and changes made based on the data. Was there the desired, positive change in an outcome, based on the change made the previous year? Accreditation and regulatory agencies want to see continuous improvement, based on evidence from outcome assessments.

Example: The nursing faculty are pleased with the increasing pass rate on the NCLEX-RN licensing exam over the last three years. The board of nursing requires that a minimum of 76% of the graduates each year (12 months) pass the exam. The national pass rate is about 87%. The faculty wanted to be above that rate. Three years ago, the pass rate was 85%, the next year it was 88%, and the most recent pass rate was

92%. The faculty looked back on the outcome data for the last three years and identified three changes that contributed to the success:

- They had a faculty workshop to improve the course exams. The exams mirror the types of questions on the NCLEX-RN exam;
- The primary textbooks they selected have additional on-line resources and sites for students and are required to be used in course assignments;
- Standardized tests for each course are taken online, similar to the NCLEX-RN exam, and students receive feedback with rationale and may retake different forms of the exam for continued practice.

A challenge is to determine which changes actually contributed to improving outcomes and how they were put in place. Prioritizing what really needs to be done, what is possible to do, and determining whether small changes can make a big difference are significant decisions.

STRUCTURE FOR USING DATA FOR PROGRAM IMPROVEMENT

All the data should be reviewed and compared with the desired outcomes. It is always interesting to see where improvements are needed. With a prioritized list, the next examination of the data can be matched to the priorities. When there are several sources of data, it is good to determine whether there is congruence among them.

Example: When the failure rate in one course is 40% higher than in other nursing courses, all the data are reviewed. This includes course evaluations, examinations, student comments, focus group at the end of the class, individual student complaints to the course leader, and comparison with grades from the previous course. It may be possible to relate the problem to one source, but it could be difficult. The examinations were changed, based on student complaints about questions and faculty desire to include more questions for content they covered. This is the only major change, so it is most likely a significant contributing factor. The faculty examined the item analysis of each exam and found problems in many questions.

When several changes are made during an academic year, it is more difficult and all areas may need to be considered. New faculty teaching the course, a new text, part of the course was online for the first time, and feedback not given in a timely manner may all contribute to poor course outcomes.

An observation: Making several changes during a short time, such as an academic year, makes it difficult to determine the outcomes that contribute to positive or negative changes. Billings and Halstead (2005) discuss intervening variables that also impact outcomes. Examples are qualification of students, preparation of students to take exams, study sessions, or student anxiety. It is complex to determine which changes actually support positive outcomes.

Decisions are made about which changes from the previous assessment, if any, contributed to the current outcomes. The current data are then compared to determine the changes from one or more prior assessments so as to trend the outcomes. Trending provides a broader picture of what has happened and what should/could be done to continuously improve. After reviewing 3 years of data, the information is summarized and the actions determined. Generally, three action choices are made:

- **Development** refers to providing new information. This could be developing a handbook, preparing instructional materials, and adding materials to courses;
- **Maintenance** indicates that the outcomes met or exceeded the established benchmarks. No changes are made in the processes, materials, or resources. For example, the BSN program received support for additional-skills lab space and equipment. The lab is state of the art and has all the new equipment needed for the BSN program;
- **Revision** requires improving, expanding, or updating materials, resources, faculty, and the environment. Changes in standards, guidelines, policies, and best practices also require that revisions are made.

Once decisions are made about which changes from the previous assessment, if any, contributed to the current outcomes, then decisions about which changes to make for the next cycle can be determined. The best scenario is to see a clear pattern in the trends.

Example: Increasing the BSN program admission grade point average (GPA) by 1.0 point each year for the past three years has resulted in reduced attrition in the first nursing course. The admission GPA went from 75% to 76%, then to 77%. Three years ago the attrition was 50%, it then dropped to 40%, and this year to 30%. Although there may be additional reasons, the change in GPA requirement could be a major factor.

The results of the comprehensive outcome assessment need to be widely shared. Different audiences and stakeholders need the information that they require and is of interest to them.

SHARING OUTCOMES

Academic and other settings usually have computer services and processes to generate reports. The individual results from exams, surveys, and other sources are compiled and summarized. When the data are kept in a central location, it can be accessed and put in different reports.

Example: The university computer center stores most of the outcome-assessment data. Faculty have access to a report with individual scores and the item analysis of each question. They also receive summarized data for their course evaluations. Student names are not shown on the results, but the number of responses on the scale is listed. Additionally, the software program can read comments and insert them in the course evaluation summary. Faculty track their individual trends in the courses they teach and use the outcome information as part of their annual performance review. The information is kept on the server and different reports can be generated when requested. Individuals and the program can print out any report they want for their own files.

Quantitative information can be organized and summarized electronically. There is software to help organize qualitative data, but the essence of it may be lost. Original comments from learners, employees, and anyone who receives or provides services can be used for several purposes. For example, highlighting positive experiences, descriptions of how a life was changed, and satisfaction with services provide another perspective on the organization. Qualitative data also provide information that is not included in structured data-collection instruments.

Example: The nursing faculty who serve on the university marketing/recruitment committee want to collect qualitative statements and use them in a variety of ways. Students and graduates who have participated in focus groups are contacted to determine whether they would like to share their experiences. Several individuals respond and a meeting is scheduled. The purpose of the project is explained. Consent forms are completed, pictures are taken, and a video segment is also recorded. After editing the material, the pictures and videos will appear on the Website, in brochures, and other recruitment information.

Educators need results of individual assessments in addition to the aggregated data for examinations, with the types of descriptive statistics described earlier. They also need summaries of all the program data in order to participate in the decision making about changes.

Example: The nursing faculty receive reports after each exam. The report lists individual student results, as well as highest and lowest scores, median, mean, item discrimination, item difficulty, standard deviation, test reliability, and standard error of measurement. (Consult a statistics text or other resources for additional statistical information.)

Administrators and leaders need to see the big picture and have access to all the data. It is helpful to have a report or executive summary to share how specific outcomes from your program/course met both the program/course and the organizational benchmarks.

Example: The dean decided to use an executive summary (described in chapter 2) to share essential pieces of information with the university leaders. She focused on the university goals of attrition, diversity of the student body, and scores on the university exit exam. She formatted the areas under each of the university goals. The information indicated university goals and benchmarks, school of nursing outcomes, and a comment. Table 6.4 presents an example of relating program goals to organizational goals.

External stakeholders need summarized reports related to specific areas. Leaders in the clinical sites are interested in summarized responses from the staff who worked with new graduates of the program. The survey would include how prepared the graduates were for practice. Student surveys of their clinical experiences at all the sites help the organization make improvements in students' experiences. Summarized reports for each agency should be developed and include qualitative responses as appropriate. Agencies can have an end of rotation or academic year meeting with faculty to discuss the students' experiences from their perspectives.

Table 6.4

CONGRUENCE OF UNIVERSITY AND PROGRAM GOALS

UNIVERSITY GOAL	BENCHMARK	BSN NURSING OUTCOME	COMMENTS
Attrition Reduce attrition in the University by 5% each year.	The University overall attrition will be 25% each year.	The overall nursing program attrition has decreased from 32% 3 years ago to 25% this year.	The nursing program will continue its current efforts to decrease attrition and review specific problem areas to further decrease it.
Diversity Increase diversity in the student body by 3% each year.	The University overall student body diversity will be 18% each year.	The overall nursing program student body diversity has increased from 10% 3 years ago to 12% this year.	The nursing program will continue to expand their efforts to attract and retain students from diverse backgrounds. New initiatives supported by the University will be implemented.
Exit exam 95% of students in their last semester will pass the required university exit exam.	The students must earn a minimum of 80% on the standardized exam.	In 2008–09, 95% of the nursing students passed the exit exam with a mean score of 97%. This is an increase of 2% over the 2 previous years.	Nursing program faculty will review results and determine which students did not pass the university exit exam and compare the scores with the standardized nursing exam scores. Students will be required to attend nursing and university study sessions.

NLCEX-RN pass rates and accreditation status are very important to clinical agencies. It is also useful to highlight how the improvements from the previous year improved the program and what will be done in the next year. Stakeholders appreciate knowing what is happening in the program and the efforts being made to improve it.

Example: The same format used in Table 6.4 is used for summarizing the selected outcomes. The information for the clinical agencies focuses on student, agency, and faculty comments about experiences and outcomes such as the NCLEX-RN pass rate.

Advisory groups need access to more detailed information than leaders in clinical agencies because they actively participate in curriculum development, implementation, and evaluation. An advisory group probably will include leaders, but will also have members from the community, and perhaps consultants. They need to review all the reports and work with the program to find solutions to issues identified in the outcome-assessment plan.

Example: Professor Jones and the dean decide to share the updated outcome-assessment plan with the advisory group. That format would allow them to see the changes over time. The document is fairly long, but the information is presented in a table, so it is easy to look at specific areas.

Students need to know the strengths and areas for improvement. They also need to know that their evaluations and comments were reviewed and taken seriously. Summaries of specific areas such as the NCLEX-RN pass rate and positive comments from students are appreciated. Students will accept and feel positive about changes being made if they know their comments are part of the rationale.

Example: Students noted that classrooms are crowded, lighting is poor, students use cell phones during class, and classes start and end late. The faculty reviewed the comments. The dean reviewed the use of the two largest classrooms and shifted times for the next semester so crowding would be reduced. Improvements in lighting were requested. Both the program faculty and student handbooks have policies about starting and ending class on time and the use of cell phones. This problem was discussed at the faculty meeting. Some faculty did not want to start class on time because there were always a few students who were late and it was disruptive. Faculty who started class on time did not allow students who were late to come into the classroom until there was a break. In those classes, students were generally on time.

The use of cell phones during class is banned. Students who used their phones were told to end their conversation and put their phones on the faculty desk. If students did this a second time, they were not allowed to bring their phones into the classroom and had to leave them in the program office. The faculty agreed to expand the policies and revise the handbooks. When focus groups were held at the end of the next semester, students were asked about the changes in the policies and whether they were actually being implemented. Most responses were positive. They appreciated the changes and the decrease in distractions. A few students were concerned about getting emergency calls. They were reminded that the student handbook suggested that family members have the student's schedule so they know when the student is in class or in clinical practicum. Students could also leave the program office phone number for anyone to call and a staff person would find them.

It is evident that the entire process requires a great deal of time and attention. It is a relief to have completed a cycle that resulted in accreditation of the program and/or the institution. Everyone may feel they are done. Actually, it is just the beginning of the process. Efforts are needed to continue the assessment processes to demonstrate continuous quality improvement.

MAINTAINING CONTINUOUS QUALITY IMPROVEMENT

In academic institutions, student data are collected at the end of each course and semester. Other areas of assessment can be reviewed at the end of the academic year. It is essential to maintain all the raw data in addition to aggregated data. Individual students' progress and their actual written work should be preserved until they graduate and become licensed or certified. If there are any questions when students fail a course or the program, the complete information may be used to review and explain what happened. It may be challenging to store the information if it cannot be done electronically. Secure cabinets and space are needed to store these items. For accreditation reviews, the evaluators will want to see the raw data and will look at selected samples of learners' work.

When there is a specific problem with assessments, it is possible to make changes. Example: On one unit exam in the nursing research course, 90% of the students had wrong answers on questions. The faculty team reviewed the questions and found typographical errors and wording that caused confusion. They corrected the problems and students did as expected the next semester.

Observation: The problem may be with the wording in the stem or in the distracters. Perhaps the content was not covered in class or the assigned learning resources. Resist the temptation to make major changes based on student or faculty opinions or likes/dislikes. Use an approach based on data from different sources, over at least one academic year.

Developing a simple, consistent method to organize and review raw data is essential for maintaining continuous quality improvement. In academic and other educational settings, it is common to take notes of meetings. These notes can also serve as a method to organize outcome data. The meeting notes can be set up with the following headings:

- **Topic**—Relate the topic to a specific element of outcome assessment, for example, critical thinking. Include the definition of the concept or area being discussed;
- **Discussion**—Describe the specific information presented, such as the tool used, results, and comparison with a benchmark. Also include information from the previous two years to compare with current results;
- **Actions**—Share what was decided by the group, what actions will be taken, and who is responsible for carrying out the actions.

In academic settings, there are different levels at which decisions are made. It is efficient if the decisions begin at the course level. For example, the community health faculty team can review test results, use the same testing format, and recommend actions. The final decision may be made by the school curriculum committee or the faculty as a whole. The notes from groups are merged, so there is one set for each area of review. Table 6.5 presents a sample of meeting notes (Anema, Brown, & Stringfield, 2003).

The purpose is to have one set of notes that has all the outcome-assessment information that needs to fit into the comprehensive plan. Responsibility for each area of information is divided among the faculty. The groups can be subcommittees of an overall curriculum committee or whatever fits into the organizational structure.

Table 6.5

BSN PROGRAM OUTCOME NOTES

BSN Program Outcome Notes
Topic: Critical Thinking—Definition: The intellectual process of actively conceptualizing, synthesizing, and evaluating.

YEAR	DISCUSSION	ACTION
2006–2007	Faculty reviewed the results of the standardized exam for Community Health. One section measured critical thinking. The benchmark was 90% of the students would have scores of 70 or above. The results ($N = 50$) showed that 88% (44) of the students had scores above 70 and 20 of the 44 students had scores above 80.	The faculty agreed they would continue without any changes because the benchmark was almost met the first time. The community health faculty team wanted to review the scores of students who scored below 70 to determine their weak areas.
2007–2008	Faculty reviewed the results of the standardized exam for Community Health. One section measured critical thinking. The benchmark was 90% of the students would have scores of 70 or above. The results showed that 92% of the students had scores above 70 and 35 of the 50 students had scores above 80.	Faculty reported they had reviewed the overall academic achievement levels of the student who had 70 the previous year. Those students had marginal scores on many exams. Specific tutorials were set up for each course. The faculty agreed they would continue without any changes because the benchmark was met this year, with more scores above 80 than the previous year.
2008–2009	Faculty reviewed the results of the standardized exam for Community Health. One section measured critical thinking. The benchmark was 90% of the students would have scores of 70 or above. The results showed that 95% of the students had scores above 70 and 40 of the 55 students had scores above 80.	The faculty agreed they would continue without any changes because the benchmark was met this year, with more scores above 80 than the previous year. After one more year of data, the faculty will discuss raising the benchmark score.

Adapted from Anema et al. (2003)

At the end of each academic year or other cycle, the new assessment information is added and the oldest is not included. Each set of notes should include the last three years. It is easy to review older outcome data because they are part of the previous permanent records, so it is still possible to look at all the outcome data from the earliest to the current.

It does take time to keep all the essential data organized and reviewed. But it takes much more time trying to find and reconstruct the outcome data at a later time. Faculty and administrative staff know how much time and effort goes into finding previous data, reviewing it, and making sense of it a few years later. Evaluators are concerned when there are gaps and missing data in self-studies and other reports. Selecting a structure for collecting outcome-assessment information supports continuous quality improvements.

Example: Professor Jones and the administrative assistant updated the course and program notes so there is a place for the new data. At the end of an academic year, the faculty can fill in the new data and report them at the last BSN faculty meeting. If there is any missing data, they can be added. Professor Jones is committed to ensuring the entire outcome data needed for the comprehensive plan are organized, aggregated, and placed in the plan. She updates the plan so it is current. The raw data are locked in file drawers in Ms. Moore's office. The data are organized by year, standards, and outcome-assessment elements. The course standardized test to measure critical thinking is organized with all the raw data and the summary report. A section is set up for the current year for all the outcome measures. Selected written materials that are part of outcome assessment are also included. Five samples of written assignments are selected for each outcome assessment. The remainder of the written materials is placed in the individual student folders. The meeting notes and comprehensive plan are also in the current year file drawer.

Information stored on the university server or on disks is identified and listed so anyone would know where to find it. Accreditation site visitors will be given limited access to university and BSN program sites, and also flash drives with selected information so they can start to review before they come on campus.

SUMMARY

Once there is a commitment to competency-based education, the most important question is, how do we know the learners are competent?

Exhibit 6.1

Consider:	Determine whether your organization has an existing plan. Use the elements that fit with the outcomes of interest. For example, if patient satisfaction, benchmarks for patient outcomes, or student retention rates are elements already being collected, fit your program/course into those elements.
	Review requirements found in regulations, standards, and guidelines to determine what is essential to your program/course.
	Assess the technology support for data collection, analysis, and reporting in your organization and determine what is possible. Is using an Excel® or other program the best way to save data? What other options are available?
	Develop a format for your comprehensive outcome-assessment plan. Use Table 6.1 as a guide.
Add information to your plan:	Identify the major regulation, standard, or guideline. State what it is, define what it means in your setting, and identify the expected outcome(s) for that element.
	Briefly describe how each outcome is being assessed (instrument, indicator, etc.).
	Indicate who is responsible or who is delegated to collect, analyze, summarize, and share the data.
	Include the frequency of assessment.
	Describe the assessment method (exam, survey, focus group, observation, etc., using rubrics).
	Provide support that the assessment method is valid, reliable, or specific for what is being assessed. If you are using a new method, discuss that reliability will be established after repeated uses. Validity of new instruments can be established by experts who can judge face or content validity. If a method has been specifically developed to measure an outcome, then discuss that process. If a nationally standardized method, such as pass rates on licensing exams is used, the validity and reliability statistics are available.
	Specify who receives the outcomes reports, usually will be more than one person.
	The last column of the plan is essential to indicate how the data were used for continuous quality improvement. It is sometimes called, "closing the loop." Imagine if you did all the work up to this point, and then never acted on what you knew from the data. In the past, this is what happened with information. It was collected and it was not used to make changes.

(continued)

Exhibit 6.1 *(continued)*

> Changes were made to educational programs based on how things were always done, intuition, personal preferences, and a trial and error approach. Although the process may not be as extensive or comprehensive as desired, the process will highlight that and then changes can be made. For example, learners complain that the texts and other learning resources are not useful or are outdated. The data can support requests for additional funding from the institution or grants. Selecting texts that have additional online resources is not costly.
>
> Look at the format to make sure you can extract segments of data for different reports.
>
> Try to maintain your format for at least three years so the data are the same and comparisons can be made for that time period.

It is easy to assess individual learner competency. It is equally important to know that the learners, as a group, have demonstrated competence. Aggregating the data provides that information. The elements of a program also must be examined to determine whether desired outcomes are being achieved.

A comprehensive outcome-assessment plan can provide that data. The desired outcomes for learners are that they can actually manage their health, function as a health care professional, and carry out the roles and responsibilities required for leadership and other positions. External groups require quality in health care organizations and educational programs. Matching assessments to desired outcomes provides the data needed to determine outcomes. The data also provide evidence to develop, revise, and maintain what is done.

The transition to competency-based education requires that the desired outcomes, not only for learners, but also for the entire program, are established. This should be done concurrently with the other steps described in the earlier chapters.

A well-constructed comprehensive outcome-assessment plan presents all the essential data to support the quality of all aspects of the program and the continuous improvement measures. The plan provides an excellent guide to what is currently being done and what needs to be done. Plans may be simple or fairly complex, depending on the scope of the program, the organizational/instructional structure, and the required external standards, regulations, and guidelines.

CHAPTER 6 ACTIVITY

The information from the previous chapters and the activities you completed are the foundation for developing a comprehensive outcome-assessment plan for your program/course. Use Exhibit 6.1 to develop your own comprehensive outcome-assessment plan.

REFERENCES

American Psychological Association. (2001). *Publication manual of the American Psychological Association* (5th ed.). Washington, DC: Author.

Anema, M. G., Brown, B. E., & Stringfield, Y. N. (2003). Organizing and presenting program outcome data. *Nursing Education Perspectives, 24*(6), 306–310.

Billings, D. M., & Halstead, J. A. (2005). *Teaching in nursing: A guide for faculty.* St. Louis, MO: Elsevier Saunders.

Houser, J. (2008). *Nursing research: Reading, using, and creating evidence.* Sudbury, MA: Jones and Bartlett.

ADDITIONAL RESOURCES

The Commission on Collegiate Nursing Education (CCNE)
Accrediting body for baccalaureate and graduate degree nursing programs.
http://www.aacn.nche.edu/Accreditation/

The Joint Commission on Accreditation of Health Care Organization (JCAHO) Accrediting body for diverse health care organizations. Provides additional information and services for quality improvements.
http://www.jointcommission.org/

The National Commission for Health Education Credentialing, Inc. (NCHEC) Accrediting body for health educators.
http://www.nchec.org/aboutnchec/about.htm

The National Certification Board for Diabetes Educators Accrediting body for diabetes educators.
http://www.ncbde.org/

The National League for Nursing Accrediting body for all levels of nursing education. Also provides certification for nurse educators.
http://www.nln.org/FacultyCertification/index.htm

Physical Therapy Licensing Accrediting body for physical therapists.
http://www.allalliedhealthschools.com/faqs/ptlicensing
University of Minnesota—Office of Measurement Services (OMS) The Descriptive Statistics Report produced by OMS gives the statistical characteristics of the test scores for a class. All the information that has been drawn from the list of scores is available, but what the scores show is hard to understand from the complete list, especially if the number of scores is large. Summary statistics provide a more comprehensible picture.
http://oms.umn.edu/oms/fce/understandingresults/descriptivesta tistics.php

7 Making the Change to CBE

JANICE L. McCOY
MARION G. ANEMA

OVERVIEW

This chapter discusses the need for change in current educational processes. Continuing to do more of the same, or making small changes, has not improved student learning outcomes or demonstrated that learners have the essential competencies to function in life and work.

The theories and principles of systems, change, and diffusion of innovation are examined in the context of their impact on educational and organizational systems, the people within those systems, and why it is important to have a well-founded basis for making changes.

Implementing competency-based education (CBE) requires a change in philosophy, expectations, and all aspects of educational and training activities. For anyone who is courageous enough to make the change, anticipating potential barriers and planning how to overcome them is essential.

INTRODUCTION

With all the information presented about CBE, it may seem like an overwhelming task to change to a new process. Many would question why they should take on all the work to make the change. Increasing emphasis is being placed on outcomes, and these outcomes are a product of behaviors designed to meet individual or organizational performance requirements. In a competency-based system, outcomes are not measured as a function of group behaviors, because in a competency-based system, each individual is expected to demonstrate 100% of all competencies required for the situation. The public and regulatory agencies are demanding accountability; using the outcome process can demonstrate competency of critical and essential behaviors. Demonstrating competency should be the goal in nursing education, continuing competence, and consumer education. A closer look at some of the reasons to support the change to a CBE system is warranted.

IS THERE A PROBLEM?

When the current processes for teaching and assessing learning are critically and thoughtfully examined, do the resulting performance outcomes still fall short of expectations? Are employers complaining that graduates are not prepared for the workplace? Do employees perform below expectation? Are patients unable to perform self-care activities to maintain or improve health? When minor changes are made to the teaching and assessment process, do the performance outcomes remain inadequate? Are educators, employers, consumers, or patient advocates questioning what is being taught because learners' behavior does not demonstrate desired performance expectations? If the answer is "yes" to any of these questions, take note that serious attention must be given to the current processes, and consideration for changing to a CBE method may be warranted.

Brown's (1983, p. 68) definition of insanity, "doing the same thing, over and over again, but expecting different results" sums up the way nursing education, continued competence, and consumer education is delivered. Although doing the same thing over and over and expecting different results may not define insanity, it may express denial about the current processes used. Change needs to occur in order to achieve the desired performance behaviors of all learners.

WHY IT IS IMPORTANT

CBE has been in the literature for more than 20 years, yet little movement has occurred toward changing to such a system. Currently, a gap exists between intentions and actions, but the interest in competencies and measuring specific learning is accelerating throughout the world.

Education

Many faculty view the movement to a competency-based system as being prescriptive, and that academic freedom will be compromised. Although institutions measure outcomes, they usually refer to retention, graduation, and placement rates. The measured outcomes are not direct measures of what students are able to do. Currently, faculty organizes courses around content and not competencies. Program outcomes, educational objectives, or learner outcomes are usually written as goal statements, which are often stated in broad, ambiguous terms. As currently written, they do not provide sufficient direction about the desired levels of learner achievement. Competency statements would create a clear, unambiguous expectation of learner performance.

Today, assessments are based on academic programs where course-based assessments are dominated by the professional judgment of individual faculty. In contrast, competency-based learning models rely on the judgments of those external to the learning process, and employ assessment strategies that are based on units of analysis that are smaller and more easily addressed than those used to assess traditional courses (Voorhees, 2001).

Using competency statements and smaller learning units permit the learner to return to one or more competencies that have not been mastered, rather than repeat the entire course. With competency-based learning, faculty is freed from the burden of defending learning outcomes that are verified only by professional judgment.

Competency-based learning also has the potential to shift the responsibility of learning from faculty to learners. Within a competency-based system, learners must assume responsibility and accountability for their own learning. Learners become active in the learning process, which is consistent with adult learning principles.

Many employers complain that new graduates do not have the ability to perform to workplace expectations. Where integration of knowledge and skills into practice settings is the desired performance, new graduates are unable to perform to expectations. This situation results in employer disappointment, new graduate frustration, and consumer displeasure. CBE can improve the match between curriculum and employment opportunities.

Continuing Competence

The competency of health care providers is crucial to providing the best possible patient care. Studies about workplace satisfaction indicate that working with competent employees increases workplace satisfaction. Alspach (2008) identified several studies supporting how critical competent providers are to high-quality patient care:

■ The Joint Commission expects health care facilities to provide care that is safe, reliable, and appropriate (The Joint Commission, 2007). Without competent staff, this expectation is difficult to meet;

■ The number-one attribute identified by staff nurses related to a satisfying work environment was having clinically competent peers (Schmalenberg & Kramer, 2008);

■ Using the essential magnet program attributes of a healthy work environment, staff nurses considered clinically competent peers in their work unit as most important (Schmalenberg & Kramer, 2008);

■ The Institute of Medicine suggests the integration of five core competencies be required to reduce the error rate (Greiner & Knebel, 2003);

■ Optimal care is achieved when patients' needs are matched to core competencies necessary to meet those needs (American Association of Critical Care Nurses, n.d.);

■ Assurance of a nurse's competence reflects the profession's responsibility to protect the public (American Nurses Association, 2007).

Because being deemed competent is so important, there is an increased demand for certifications of competencies that are not being met by traditional higher educational providers. These certifications are built to meet specific industry demands, and are based solely on the learners' ability to demonstrate that specific competencies have been achieved.

Consumer Education

Significant changes are occurring in the health care delivery system, and more changes will occur as the health care system is redefined and restructured. Change can be seen as a constant as the nation struggles with providing high-quality health care to all at an affordable cost:

■ Care is shifting from acute care facilities to the community, thus requiring consumers to actively participate in the care of self or of family members. Across the United States, patients and family members are assuming many of the health care provider roles traditionally performed by health care providers. CBE, with its focus on essential behaviors, would clarify expectations of caregivers;

■ Access to the Internet has provided vast amounts of health care information to consumers. Many consumers search the Internet before seeking a health care provider. Although this practice may reduce the number of unnecessary visits, it may also delay visits where early intervention is warranted. Consumers' competency in Internet search strategies, and how to identify factual health information/practices, is increasing in importance;

■ The older population is growing, and with this growth comes an increased need to manage chronic illness. Management of chronic illness strives to maintain or improve well-being. When chronic illness is properly managed, entry into more costly health care situations can be reduced. Management of chronic illness requires the consumer to be actively involved in self-care. The volume of information about specific chronic illness can be overwhelming to an older individual. With CBE's focus on essential behaviors, information overload can be controlled.

As changes occur in health care delivery processes, consumers of all ages are being asked to assume increased responsibility for maintaining or improving personal health. To accomplish this, consumers must be active participants in their own health care. This can be problematic for patient educators because of the diverse expectations of consumers. There is a segment of the population that still wants to be taken care of, with health care decisions being made by the health care providers. This population is not interested in assuming responsibility for health decisions or for being accountable for personal practices. CBE may not change the outcomes for this population, because it does not choose to become competent. Choosing competence requires commitment to making changes in order to achieve expected outcomes. Sometimes consumers choose to not commit to changing personal behavior. CBE will not help these individuals. Given limited available resources, one must consider whether consumers unwilling to change personal behaviors will result in higher health care costs without achieving the desired and expected outcomes.

COMMITMENT TO CHANGE

Based on the changing expectations in education, workplace requirements, continuing competence, and consumer responsibilities, the environment is ripe for change. Making the commitment to change to a CBE system will meet the demands of multiple stakeholders. However, making the commitment to change will require strong resolve and determination. The decision to change to a competency-based process should not be taken lightly, for it will require thoughtful, critical analysis of the essential behaviors necessary to achieve desired outcomes. It will also require changes in the way competence is measured. With the increased emphasis on objective measurement of outcomes, the evaluation process will need extensive revisions. The traditional repetitive-process assessment and the use of multiple lists of skill check-offs will no longer be appropriate (Bargagliotti, Luttrel, & Lenburg, 1999). Changing the assessment of competence may result in increased anxiety about the change and resistance to the change, but when stakeholders play a central role in the decision process and understand the logic driving the change, they frequently become motivated to change the process quickly (Bargagliotti, Luttrel, & Lenburg, 1999). An understanding of theories on change, diffusion of innovation, and systems will ease the transition to competency-based learning.

STRATEGIES TO SUPPORT CBE INITIATIVES

The implementation of a new or different way of thinking and approaching education requires strategic planning. Knowing what to expect, and ensuring the initial efforts are positive, requires looking at the impact on the entire organization, the people involved, and the resources. Three theories are especially useful: systems, change, and diffusion of innovation.

Systems Theory

Systems theory focuses on changes that happen because of the interactions within a situation or organization. General systems theory helps to understand how the functions of parts influence the whole system, organization, program, or patent/client. The subsystems are affected by changes and inputs of the others. Systems change because of inputs. Change within a system requires a change in balance. There is feedback, which goes to the system inputs to determine the impact (Hood & Leddy, 2003). Educators need to anticipate the system impact on any change in one part.

Clancy, Effken, and Pesut (2008) examined the application of complex systems theory to nursing education, research, and practice. The complexity of health care and educational systems is well known. A complex system (CS) has some of the following characteristics:

- There are highly connected networks of components from which high-level behaviors (e.g., physical objects, people, or groups of people) come forward.
- Research in the transdisciplinary field of CS, using modeling and simulation to analyze CS behavior, helps to understand common behaviors, regardless of the discipline.
- An example of an application of CS principles is the use of computer simulation to determine the benefits and drawbacks of new procedures, protocols, and practices before having to actually implement them. In educational settings, the inclusion of new computational tools and their applications in nursing education is also gaining attention.
- Education in complex systems and applied computational applications has been endorsed by the Institute of Medicine, the American Organization of Nurse Executives, and the American Association of Colleges of Nursing as essential training of nurse leaders.

Application of Systems Theory

The University of Kansas School of Nursing provides an example of the use of systems theory in nursing education. It has adopted a modified systems theory as the organizing framework for the construction and implementation of the nursing curricula:

- Four major concepts with definitional statements and sub-concepts comprise the elements of the system. The major concepts are client systems, environment, health, and nursing;
- The systems framework supports a commitment to teach students theory and research-based humanistic nursing practice, focused on health, wellness and illness of client systems of varying complexity, within a rapidly changing health care delivery system;
- The rapid evolution of nursing science, practice, and education demands on-going reexamination of categories and concepts. Program revision includes using systems theory to make changes in the curricula. Data are collected and used to improve the programs. The University of Kansas School of Nursing Philosophy. (Available at: *http://www2.kumc.edu/son/vorientation/concept.html*)

Considering the elements of systems theory when implementing CBE is essential. The impact on the entire system is significant. Resources are needed to make the change. Faculty, students, staff, and external stakeholders need to understand how CBE can improve program and course outcomes and what is needed to accomplish them. Although systems theory is useful in looking at the total picture to make sure a major change is possible, change theory provides a guide for how to implement a change such as CBE.

Change Theory

Change theory addresses the impact of change on individuals and groups. Emotions become a large part of a change process when people have to cope with the changes. There are different models that describe the processes. Carnall's model (1990) listed five steps to cope with change:

- Stage 1—Deny: new ideas or change are not valid;
- Stage 2—Defensive: by experiencing depression or frustration;

- **Stage 3**—Discarding: by recognizing that change is inevitable or needed;
- **Stage 4**—Adapting to change but feeling angry about it;
- Stage 5—Internalization and recognizing that the change will happen.

Anticipating that change will be difficult, and that individuals and groups will be at different stages, requires strategies to ease into the transition.

Change Strategies

There are several approaches to helping people through change. Some examples are:

- Empirical—Rational approaches are based on the concept that people respond in rational ways. Education that provides options for accepting change will be enough to encourage people to change behaviors, for example, providing training for new technology will make people accept and use it.
- Facilitative strategies include making information available and providing feedback and solutions. There have to be adequate resources, support, and follow-up to demonstrate the change is doable.
- Persuasive strategies rely on rationale, suggestion, encouragement, and use of incentives. This strategy is helpful when people are not very open to changes, and can help change attitudes and behavioral commitment.
- Power strategies may have a negative connotation, because it may seem like coercion. There may be a low level of commitment to the change because people expect negative outcomes or expect rewards. It is also necessary to continue monitoring changes in behavior.

Persons who are the leaders in implementing CBE need to be careful about the strategies they select, making sure to match them with the outcomes they desire (Hood & Leddy, 2003). The impact of change on systems and strategies to help people change does not explain why some people change, why rate of acceptance varies, and why some never change. Rogers (1964) developed and published a theory to explain these variations.

Diffusion of Innovations Theory

The Diffusion of Innovations (DoI) theory focuses on how new ideas, techniques, or processes, especially those related to technology, are accepted. Some of the points that support adopting innovations are presented:

■ Determine whether the relative advantage of the innovation is better than what currently exists. This advantage could be economic, a learning outcome, or satisfaction;
■ The consistency between existing values and practices and the proposed innovation;
■ If the innovation is simple to understand and implement, it will be adopted more quickly than one that is difficult and complex;
■ If it is possible to implement an innovation on a trial basis, people feel more comfortable with trying it;
■ Actually seeing the results of an innovation such as CBE increases the chance of adopting the innovation because of the benefits to the organization.

Communication, through different channels, flows through the organizational social systems. The stages for passing on information are:

■ **Knowledge** starts with knowing something exists and an understanding of the functions or purposes;
■ **Persuasion** relates to forming a favorable attitude toward the innovation;
■ **Decision** is making a commitment to adopting the innovation;
■ **Implementation** begins when the innovation is put into place;
■ **Confirmation** consists of reinforcement based on the positive outcomes from the innovation (Clarke, 1999).

Understanding that persons have different approaches to accepting innovations is important, because the leaders can match the strengths of individuals to the tasks that must be done to implement CBE. The rate at which people respond to change determines their placement into the following categories:

- Innovators are at the front of the line, venturesome, and ready to try new things;
- The early adopters are open to new ideas, and can cope with some uncertainty;
- The early majority are also open to change, but need to be persuaded to adopt the innovation;
- The late majority are skeptics, and will wait until they see the benefit of an innovation;
- The laggards will be actively opposed to new ideas (Nutbeam and Harris, 2001);
- The leaders responsible for implementing CBE also need to be aware of the behavioral and attitudinal responses of employees, students, and patients/clients;
- Opinion leaders have relatively frequent informal influence over the behavior of others;
- Change agents positively influence innovation decisions by mediating between the change agency and the relevant social system;
- A primary change agent can receive support from change aides who can have more intensive contact with clients. Change aides may not have the highest level of technical competence, but are seen as credible and trustworthy by others.

Implementing CBE requires attention to the elements of the three theories in order to help smooth the transition to developing and implementing CBE in educational settings.

WHAT IS NEEDED FOR CHANGE

In organizations, adopting innovations can foster resistance. Competency-based learning methods are no exception. Applying the principles and concepts of systems, change, and DoI theories can smooth the progress to competency-based learning. According to Bargagliotti, Luttrel, and Lenburg (1999), to successfully change to a potentially difficult and controversial system requires understanding not only of change, but also the influence on and significance for those affected by the change. Some areas to consider when contemplating change to a CBE process are:

■ **The organizations** (such as educational institutions and health care facilities)

Does the organization support a change to CBE? The organization must want to change and demonstrate support for the change through action. Resources need to be provided in order to develop and implement a competency-based learning system;

■ **What would be the impact on the organization?**

The organization may have to implement other changes, such as changing its philosophy about assessment of competency or changing its staff evaluation policies and processes;

■ **Do the people affected by the change understand the rationale for the change?**

People affected by the change must be able to see the benefits to implementing a competency-based learning system. The organization can conduct small focus groups to inform people about the change and provide a forum for the people to ask questions and express concerns;

■ **How will the change affect the system where the change occurs? How will the change affect other parts of the system not involved with the change directly?**

If one organizational unit changes to competency-based learning and assessment, that unit will need to learn a different way of demonstrating desired outcomes. System-wide, there could be frustration when different learning and assessment systems are in place. If the measurement standards are different, staff transfers between units may pose problems.

Looking at the overall organization situation when considering changing to a competency-based learning system is important, but nursing education, continuing competence, and consumer education have specific areas to examine:

■ Nursing Education
  ○ Will the program's foundational documents (philosophy, mission, framework, etc) need revisions?
    Revising all foundational documents will be a major undertaking for any faculty group, but the curriculum is sup-

ported by this foundation. At the very least, the program's philosophy of teaching/learning may need revision so it is consistent with CBE principles.

o Will the faculty embrace or resist a change to CBE?

Recognize and strengthen the personal values and experiences faculty bring to the learning environment. In addition, faculty must learn about the benefits and safeguards in using a competency-based approach. If there is strong commitment for making the change, identify the early adopters to get the process started.

o What will faculty need to be able to do in order to change to a competency-based system?

Introduce a model like Lenburg's COPA model (1999) to facilitate the conversion to competency-based learning. Faculty understand problem-based learning, and this process can be used to assist the faculty in the conversion to a competency-based learning system.

o Will students be resistant to the change?

Students have a vested interest in the educational process and want to be successful. They need to fully understand the expectations and processes with CBE. CBE must be presented positively and shown how it assists the students to be successful.

o Will faculty and students embrace active learning principles?

Competency-based learning uses adult learning principles that support active learning. Adult learning principles also require adults to be responsible and accountable for personal learning. Faculty have traditionally used lecture as the primary teaching method. This method fosters passive learning. Students have come to expect lecture as the primary teaching method, so changing current faculty practices and student expectations will be the challenge.

■ Continuing Competence

o Will the organization's policies and procedures (position descriptions, evaluation processes, continued employment decisions, etc.), need revisions?

Revising policies and procedures will be a major undertaking for any organization. At the very least, the policies/procedures for hiring, evaluating, and continued employment recommendations may need revision to be consistent with competency-based outcome expectations.

○ Will the staff embrace or resist a change to competency-based process?

Once again, recognize and strengthen the personal values and experiences the staff bring to the work environment. In addition, staff must learn about the benefits and safeguards to using a competency-based approach. The staff evaluates the work environment as being positive when coworkers are competent. If there is strong commitment for making the change, identify the early adopters to get the process started.

○ What will staff need to be able to do in order to change to a competency-based system?

Introduce a model like Lenburg's COPA model (1999) to facilitate the conversion to competency-based learning. Some adaptations may need to be done to the model so it fits the employment setting. Staff must be involved in identifying competencies and in developing the assessment processes to measure competence.

○ Will staff embrace a system that expects performance of essential behaviors at 100%?

Competency-based learning uses adult learning principles that require adults to be responsible and accountable for personal learning and performance. Staff may not initially embrace a competency-based system, because it requires individuals to actively demonstrate competence. Managers are more likely to embrace this system, as the measurement of competency is objective and requires achievement at 100% of essential behaviors.

■ Consumer Education

○ Consumer health-related educational materials currently available may not be using a competency-based approach, and materials providers may not choose to change to such a system.

Patient educators may choose to convert existing consumer educational materials to a competency-based method, or they may choose to develop assessments that measure a consumer's ability to perform essential behaviors.

○ Will the consumer embrace or resist a change to a competency-based process?

Consumers who assume responsibility and accountability for personal choices may be more open to a competency-based method. Resistance may be encountered by consumers who want to remain more passive or less involved with personal health care decisions.

○ What will patient educators need to be able to do in order to change to a competency-based system?

Introduce a model like Lenburg's COPA model (1999) to facilitate the conversion to competency-based learning. Some adaptations may need to be done to the model so it fits consumer education needs. Patient educators and consumers need to be involved in identifying competencies and in developing the assessment processes to measure competence.

○ Will a system that expects performance of essential behaviors at 100% be embraced?

Patient educators and other health care providers should embrace such a system, because the expected outcome is a healthier consumer population. There may be segments of the consumer population that will not embrace a change because they will be responsible and accountable for personal health decisions and health care practices. Some consumers will continue to be passive rather than active recipients in health care decisions and personal care.

SUMMARY

Current educational processes are not working; to continue to do the same thing, but expect different outcomes, is unrealistic and unacceptable. Student learning outcomes are not improving, nor are learners demonstrating the essential competencies required by employers. CBE has been in the literature for years; now is the time to embrace a learning and assessment process that promotes achievement of expected outcomes.

Theories and principles of systems change, and the Diffusion of Innovations theory can help change agents understand what is necessary to make change happen, and to plan accordingly. Understanding the

Exhibit 7.1

Is there a problem?	Select one of the issues/concerns you listed in the chapter 1 Activity.
	Explain why this is a problem for your institution/organization.
Why is it important?	Explain why this issue/concern is important to you or to your institution/organization.
	Determine whether the issue/concern is important enough to drive a change to CBE.
	Consider what the possible outcomes will be if no change is made.
	Evaluate whether the possible outcomes will be acceptable to you or your institution/organization if no change is made.
	Consider what the possible outcomes will be if change is made.
	Evaluate whether the possible outcomes are acceptable to you or your institution/organization if a change is made.
	Judge whether the possible outcomes with change are an improvement over the current outcomes.
Commitment to change	Evaluate the strength of your commitment to changing to a CBE process.
	Identify others within your institution/organization with a strong commitment to changing to a CBE process.
	Determine how to secure the commitment of the institution/organization decision makers for making the change. What is needed for change?
	Explain what you or your institution/organization need for change to occur.
	Explain how implementing a CBE system would improve outcomes in your institution/organization.
	Strategies to support CBE initiatives.
	Identify strategies that would assist you to implement a CBE course or program.

impact on educational and organizational systems, and the people within and outside of those systems, is very important. Successful change cannot occur unless educational/organizational systems and the people affected by the change are willing to be responsible and accountable for actively working toward positive change.

Implementing CBE will require many changes in educational programs, workplace practices, and other consumer learning expectations and the activities that support achievement of expectations. It takes courage to make the change, vision to spot the potential barriers, and determination to develop and implement well-thought-out plans to achieve success. The reward is being able to move forward with improved conditions, and no longer be frustrated by trying to achieve outstanding outcomes through use of the same old techniques.

CHAPTER 7 ACTIVITY

The information from the previous chapters and the activities you completed at the end of each chapter are the foundation for developing strategies for planning and implementing change in your program/ course. Use Exhibit 7.1 to help identify what needs to be done to make the change to competency-based education.

REFERENCES

American Association of Critical-Care Nurses. (n.d.). *AACN Synergy model for patient care*. Retrieved August 8, 2008, from: http://new.aacn.org/WD/Certifications/contentsynmodel.pcms?pid=1&&menu=#Basic

American Nurses Association. (2007). *Draft position statement on competence and competency*. Retrieved August 8, 2008, from: http://www.nursecredentialing.org/cert/archives/2007/CompetenceCompetencyPositionStatement.pdf.

Bargagliotti, T., Luttrel, M., & Lenburg, C. B. (1999). Reducing threats to the implementation of a competency-based performance assessment system. *Online Journal of Issues in Nursing, 4*(3). Retrieved August 8, 2009, from http://www.nursingworld.org/MainMenuCategories/ANAMarketplace/ANAPeriodicals/OJIN/TableofContents/Volume41999/

Brown, R. M. (1983). *Sudden death*. New York: Bantam Books.

Carnall, C. A. (1990). *Managing change in organizations*. New York: Prentice Hall.

Clancy, T. R., Effken, J. A., & Pesut, D. (2008). Applications of complex systems theory in nursing education, research, and practice. *Nursing Outlook, 56*(5), 248–256.

Clarke, R. (1999). *A primer in diffusion of innovations theory*. Retrieved August 8, 2009, from: http://www.rogerclarke.com/SOS/InnDiff.html

Greiner A. C., & Knebel, E. (2003). *Health professions education: A bridge to quality*. Washington, DC: National Academies Press.

Hood, L. J., & Leddy, S. K. (2003). *Conceptual bases of professional nursing*. Philadelphia: Lippincott Williams Wilkins.

Joint Commission on Accreditation of Healthcare Organizations. (2007). *Assessing Hospital Staff Competence*. Oakbrook Terrace, IL: Joint Commission Resources.

Lenburg, C. B. (1999). The framework, concepts, and methods of the competency outcomes and performance assessment (COPA) model. *Online Journal of Issues in Nursing, 4*(3). Retrieved December 15, 2008, from http://www.nursingworld.org/ojin

Nutbeam, D., & Harris, E. (2001). *Theory in a nutshell: A guide to health promotion theory*. Roseville, NSW, Australia: McGraw-Hill.

Rogers, E.M. (1964). *Diffusion of innovations* (3rd ed.). New York: The Free Press.

Schmalenberg, C., & Kramer, M. (2008). Clinically competent peers and support for education: Structures and practices that work. *Crit Care Nurse*. 28(4), 54–65.

ADDITIONAL RESOURCE

Change Theory: The Motivation it Gives to Health Care Nursing *http://www.en.articles-gratuits.com/change-theory-the-motivation-it-gives-to-health-care-nursing-id374.php*

Appendix:
Additional Resources

JANICE L. McCOY
MARION G. ANEMA

The resources in this Appendix provide additional information and examples of the use of CBE in various settings.

Chapter 1 Vision of Competency-Based Education

TAFE NSW. New South Wales Department of Education and Training. Competency Based Training.
http://www.icvet.tafensw.edu.au/resources/competency_based.htm

The site includes links to CBE sites and other resources for training and education in Australia.

From the TASE NSW Website: Competency-based training (CBT) is an approach to vocational education and training that places emphasis on what a person can do in the workplace as a result of completing a program of training. Competency standards are industry-determined specifications of performance that set out the skills, knowledge, and attitudes required to operate effectively in a specific industry or profession. Competency standards are made up of units of competency, which are themselves made up of elements of competency, together with performance criteria, a range of variables, and an evidence guide. Competency standards are an endorsed component of a training package.

University of Minnesota–Duluth. Transferable Skills Survey.
http://www.d.umn.edu/kmc/career_transfer_survey.html

The University of Minnesota–Duluth has a survey for graduates to rate their skills in the areas of communication, research and planning, human relations, organization, leadership, and management, and work survival.

Educational Testing Service (ETS).
http://www.ets.org

ETS, a nonprofit institution, has a mission to advance quality and equity in education for all people worldwide.

From the ETS Website: We help teachers teach, students learn, and parents measure the educational and intellectual progress of their children. We do this by:

- Listening to educators, parents and critics;
- Learning what students and their institutions need;
- Leading in the development of new and innovative products and services.

Watch a video: *"Positioning Educational Assessment for the 21st Century"*

Read a report: *"What Does It Mean to be an Educational Measurement Organization in the 21st Century"*

Our Mission: To advance quality and equity in education by providing fair and valid assessments, research, and related services. Our products and services measure knowledge and skills, promote learning and educational performance, and support education and professional development for all people worldwide.

Student Learning Outcomes: Amid calls for greater accountability in higher education, ETS is helping the postsecondary community examine, define, and evaluate strategies for creating an evidence-based assessment system for student learning.

HealthStream Learning Center. Healthstream Competency Compass. *http://www.healthstream.com/Products/*

From the HealthStream Learning Center Website: Competency Compass™ is an online competency assessment and performance management system designed to assist hospital personnel with competency mapping and educational planning.

Chapter 2 Developing and Applying Competency-Based Education

North Carolina State University Internet Resources for Higher Education Outcomes Assessment. *http://www2.acs.ncsu.edu/UPA/assmt/resource.htm*

This site indicates new resources, lists of links, and new pages on individual institutions' assessment programs.

Calhoun, J, G., Vincent, E. T., Baker, G. R., Butler, P. W., & Chen, S. L. (2004). **Competency identification and modeling in healthcare leadership.** *Journal of Health Administration Education, 21*(4), 419–140.

From the abstract: In line with the current interest in leadership development across many industries today, a number of competency-based educational programming initiatives have been launched in professional education. The National Summit on the Future of Education and Practice in Health Management and Policy in 2001 called for the documentation of learning outcomes for continual educational improvement in health management and policy.

Cowan, D. T., Norma, I., & Coopamah, V. P. (2007). **Competence in nursing practice: A controversial concept: A focused review of literature.** *Accident and Emergency Nursing, 15*(1), 20–26.

From the abstract: The competency-based approach to education, training, and assessment has surfaced as a key policy in industrialized nations. Following the transition of nurse preparation to the higher education sector, the need to attenuate the tension of interests between employer and educator arose. Although the competency-based approach has the potential to fulfill this, the application of competence to nursing is controversial and little consensus exists on definition. This paper synthesizes a significant volume of literature relating to the acceptability and definition of the concept of competence with regard to nursing practice.

Chapter 3   Applying a Model to Develop and Implement a Competency-Based Education Program/Course

Council on Education for Public Health (CEPH). Competencies and Learning Objectives.
http://www.ceph.org/files/public/Competencies.pdf

From the CEPH Website: The purpose of this article is to support faculty of schools of public health/public health programs (SPH/PHP) as they consider approaches and make decisions for competency-based program planning and curriculum development. This document is provided for assistance, and does not intend to prescribe a process for curriculum development. It will provide an introduction to the concepts and references to support continued examination of these issues.

University of MA—Boston. The College of Community and Public Service.
http://www.cpcs.umb.edu/support/studentsupport/new_student/competency_education.htm

The site includes resources for new students who wish to understand CBE.

U.S. Department of Education Institute of Education Sciences. National Center for Education Statistics. Defining and Assessing Learning: Exploring Competency-Based Initiatives.
http://nces.ed.gov/pubSearch/pubsinfo.asp?pubid=2002159

From the Institute of Education Sciences Website: Legislators, employers, accrediting agencies, and others are often more interested in what skills and abilities students have, than in the number of credit hours the students have accumulated. This report is a hands-on resource that introduces basic information about the construction and use of competency assessments and includes the results of eight case studies of competency-based programs. A set of operating principles to guide best practices in this field is gleaned from these case studies. The publication also relays important information about the theory of competency-based education and addresses issues involved in compiling, analyzing, maintaining, and reporting data about students' competencies.

Eastern Regional Competency Based Education Consortium (ERCBEC).
http://www.ercbec.org

From the ERCBEC Website: The predominant goal for the Consortium is to hold an annual, affordable conference which offers professional development opportunities which focus on faculty and administrators' involvement in systematic planning, classroom learning, and assessment.

Bowden, John. Competency-Based Education——Neither a Panacea nor a Pariah.
http://crm.hct.ac.ae/events/archive/tend/018bowden.html

Professor John A. Bowden, Director of the Educational Programme Improvement Group, the Royal Melbourne Institute of Technology, Australia, presents an in-depth essay about the differences in perspective about CBE and its history and background.

Meretoja, R., Isoaho, H., & Leino-Kilpi, H. (2004). Nurse competence scale: Development and psychometric testing. *Journal of Advanced Nursing, 47*(2), 124–133.

From the abstract: This paper describes the development and testing of the Nurse Competence Scale, an instrument with which the level of nurse competence can be assessed in different hospital work environments.

Redfern, S., Norman, I., Calman, L., Watson, R., & Murrells, T. (2002). Assessing competence to practice in nursing: A review of the literature. *Research Papers in Education, 17*(1), 51–77.

From the abstract: Recent reforms of nursing education have led to calls for assessment of clinical performance to contribute to academic qualifications that incorporate professional awards. Questions then follow concerning the psychometric quality of methods available for assessing competence and performance, and the ability of the methods to distinguish between different levels of practice. The purpose of this review of the literature is to analyze methods of assessing competence to practice in nursing and draw conclusions on their reliability and validity. The methods reviewed include questionnaire rating scales, ratings by observation, criterion-referenced rating scales, simulations including the objective structured clinical examination (OSCE of skill acquisition), Benner's model of redirection, in and on practice, self-assessment and multimethod approaches.

Smith, A. P., & Lichtveld, M. Y. (2007). A competency-based approach to expanding the cancer care workforce. *MEDSURG Nursing*, 16(2), 109–117.

From the abstract: The Cancer Core Competency Initiative aims to bolster the basic cancer care knowledge and skills of the general health workforce. This article serves as an introduction to the initiative, including the project development methods, competency definitions, and future implementation plans.

Krumliolz, H. M., Normand, S. T., Spertus, J. A., Shahlan, D. M., & Bradley, E. H. (2007). Heart failure: The case for outcomes measurement. *Health Affairs*, 26(1), 75–85.

From the abstract: To complement the current process measures for treating patients with heart attacks and with heart failure, which target gaps in quality but do not capture patient outcomes, the Centers for Medicare and Medicaid Services (CMS) has proposed the public reporting of hospital-level 30-day mortality for these conditions in 2007. We present the case for including measurements of outcomes in the assessment of hospital performance, focusing on the care of patients with heart attacks and with heart failure. Recent developments in the methodology and standards for outcomes measurement have laid the groundwork for incorporating outcomes into performance monitoring efforts for these conditions.

Chapter 4 Transitioning to the CBE Approach

Cook, L. R., & Salveson, C. (January, 2006). Transforming RN/BS distance education: Competency-based approach using course CD-ROMs. In M. H. Oermann (Ed.), *Annual review of nursing education* (Vol. 4, pp. 103–127). New York: Springer Publishing Company.

From chapter 6: Associate-degree-educated nurses living in rural areas of Oregon experience the increasingly complex demands of nursing practice in the midst of a nursing shortage, and at the same time are confronted with barriers to accessing a baccalaureate nursing education (Northwest Health Foundation, 2001). The Oregon Health & Science University (OHSU) School of Nursing (SON) has a 35-year history of attempting to meet the challenges of a 94,000-square-mile campus and to provide access to baccalaureate (BS) nursing education for RNs throughout Oregon through its four regional campuses.

Jackson, M. (2009). *Pocket guide for patient education.* Boston: Jones and Bartlett.

From the Jones and Bartlett Website: This pocket guide contains all the patient education information front-line nurses and students need at their fingertips when on the hospital floor. This resource is made up of conversion charts, instructions, and other basic information that nurses can refer to quickly and share with patients and their families.

Zane, T. (2008). **Domain definition: The foundation of competency assessment.** *Assessment Update, 20*(1), 3-4.

From the abstract: This article details the building of a competency-based degree program beginning with competence definition activities that focus on what successful graduates need to be able to *do* and the related skills and information they need to *know*.

Chapter 5 Developing Valid and Reliable Assessments

McDonald, M. (2008). *The nurse educator's guide to assessing learning outcomes* (2nd ed). Boston: Jones and Bartlett.

This book addresses the increased pressure that the NCLEX and other certification exams are placing on nursing students and faculty. It guides classroom educators through the process of developing effective classroom exams and individual test items.

Oregon Consortium for Nursing Education (OCNE). Competency Rubrics and Benchmarks.
http://www.ocne.org/

From the OCNE Website: A rubric is an assessment tool that is designed to convey performance expectations, provide systematic feedback to students about their performance, and promote student learning.

The Curriculum Committee for the Oregon Consortium for Nursing Education (OCNE) has developed rubrics describing performance levels for each of the 10 competencies guiding the curriculum. These rubrics can be used as an assessment tool for students in either clinical practice or in simulation, in situations that require the student to demonstrate one or more competencies. The rubrics can be used alone or in combination, depending on the demands of the performance task and the level of the student.

Each rubric has several components: (a) a statement of the competency to be demonstrated; (b) a scale that describes how well or poorly the student performs during a competency demonstration; (c) dimensions that lay out the parts of the competency that are vital to successful achievement; and (d) descriptions of the dimensions at each level of performance.

Case, R. E. (2008). Independent learning and test question development: The intersection of student and content. *Assessment Update,* *20*(1), 5-7.

The article uses the Western Governors model, which requires a high degree of independence on the part of the student to master competences through independent study, exploration, and collaboration. Assessment development is explained.

Nicastro, G., & Moreton, K. M. (2008). Development of quality performance tasks at Western Governors University. *Assessment Update,* *20*(1), 8-9.

From the abstract: The article explains how to develop performance-based assessments that assess higher level cognitive skills by asking students to apply their learning in an approximation of real-world situations. The key to the development of performance-based assessments is the use of consistent terms and formats, which facilitates interrater reliability, clear instructions to students, and the development process.

Chapter 6 Data Collection and Use to Verify Achievement of Outcomes

Hager, P., Gonczi, A., & Athanasou, J. (1994). General issues about assessment of competence. *Assessment & Evaluation in Higher Education, 19*(1), 3–16.

From the abstract: In simple terms, competency-based assessment is the assessment of a person's competence against prescribed standards of performance. Thus, if an occupation has established a set of, say, entry-level competency standards, then these prescribe the standards of performance required of all new entrants to that occupation. Competency-based assessment is the process of determining whether a candidate meets the prescribed standards of performance, i.e., whether they demonstrate competence.

Taras, M. (2005). Assessment—summative and formative: Some theoretical reflections. *British Journal of Educational Studies, 53*(4), 466–478.

From the abstract: This paper attempts to clarify the definitions of the central terms relating to assessment. It argues that all assessment begins with summative assessment (which is a judgment), and that formative assessment is, in fact, summative assessment plus feedback which is used by the learner.

Kan, A. (2007). An alternative method in the new educational program from the point of performance-based assessment: Rubric scoring scales. *Educational Sciences: Theory & Practice, 7*(1), 144–152.

From the abstract: Scoring rubrics are useful to serve performance assessment for learning and assessment because they can be created for a variety of subjects and situations. Rubrics look like more suitable and effective tools for summative and formative evaluation because they include a qualitative description of the performance criteria. In recent years, rubrics have been accepted as the most popular performance-based assessment tools. It has been recommended that rubrics be used in the new educational program in Turkey, which was revised and reorganized in the scope of constructualism. It has also been stated at an annual meeting of the Ministry of Education that rubrics should be preferred for all lectures when implementing an effective performance-based assessment. However, it is not an easy procedure to develop an effective rubric. Many educational scientists have studied rubrics and their properties. This article examines the guidelines and principles from the educational literature that are related to scoring rubrics.

Swider, S., Levin, P., Ailey, S., Breakwell, S., Cowell, J., McNaughton, D., & O'Rourke, M. (2006). **Matching a graduate curriculum in public/community health nursing to practice competencies: The Rush University experience.** *Public Health Nursing, 23*(2), 190–195.

From the abstract: An evidence-based approach to Public/Community Health Nursing (P/CHN) requires that P/CHN educators prepare practitioners with the relevant skills, attitudes, and knowledge. Such education should be competency-based and have measurable outcomes to demonstrate student preparation. In 2003, the Quad Council competencies were developed to be applied at two levels of public health nursing practice: the staff nurse/generalist role and the manager/specialist/consultant role. This paper describes a process for evaluation and revision of a graduate curriculum to prepare advanced practice nurses who have the knowledge and proficiency in all relevant competencies.

Hoge, M. A., Paris, M., Adger, H., Collins, F. L., Finn, C. V., Fricks, L., et. al (2005). **Workforce competencies, in behavioral health: An overview.** *Administration and Policy in Mental Health, 32*(5/6), 593–631.

From the abstract: Competency-based training approaches are being used more in health care to guide curriculum content and ensure accountability and outcomes in the educational process. This article provides an overview of the state of competency development in the field of behavioral health. Specifically, it identifies the groups and organizations that have conducted and supported this work, summarizes their progress in defining and assessing competencies, and discusses both the obstacles and future directions for such initiatives. A major purpose of this article is to provide a compendium of current competency efforts, so that these might inform and enhance ongoing competency development in the varied behavioral health disciplines and specialties. These varied resources may also be useful in identifying the core competencies that are common to the multiple disciplines and specialties.

National Commission for Health Education Credentialing, Inc.
http://www.nchec.org/credentialing/responsibilities/

   This site includes a description of the responsibilities and competencies of health educators.

Gateway Engineering Education Coalition.
www.gatewaycoalition.org/files/Competency_Workshop.ppt

   This site provides PPT slides on the subject of developing competency-based surveys to provide students with developmental feedback on learning outcomes.

Chapter 7 Making the Change to CBE

Robinson, L. (2009). *A summary of diffusion of innovations.* Available at:
   http://www.enablingchange.com.au/Summary_Diffusion_Theory.pdf

   This article provides a quick review of the main points of the theory of diffusion of innovations.

Kritsonis, A. (2005). **Comparison of change theories.** *International Journal of Scholarly Academic Intellectual Diversity, 8*(1), 1–7.

   From the abstract: The article compares the characteristics of Lewin's Three-Step Change Theory, Lippitt's Phases of Change Theory, Prochaska and DiClemente's Change Theory, social cognitive theory, and the theory of reasoned action and planned behavior to one another. Leading industry experts will need to continually review and provide new information relative to the change process, and to our evolving society and culture.

University of Twente. *Diffusion of innovations theory.* Available at:
   http://www.cw.utwente.nl/theorieenoverzicht/

   The article provides a summary of the diffusion of innovations theory.

Teamtechnology. *Change management: Five basic principles, and how to apply them.* Available at: *http://www.teamtechnology.co.uk/change management.html*

   This article takes a look at the basic principles of change management and provides some tips on how those principles can be applied.

Bellinger, G. (2004). *Change management: The Columbo theory*. Available at: *http://www.systems-thinking.org/columbo/columbo.htm*

This essay applies systems theory to implementing and managing change.

Index